# Patient-Centered Medicine

# Patient-Centered Medicine

*A Human Experience*

David H. Rosen, MD
Uyen B. Hoang, MD

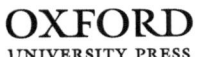

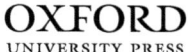
UNIVERSITY PRESS

Oxford University Press is a department of the University of Oxford. It furthers
the University's objective of excellence in research, scholarship, and education
by publishing worldwide. Oxford is a registered trade mark of Oxford University
Press in the UK and certain other countries.

Published in the United States of America by Oxford University Press
198 Madison Avenue, New York, NY 10016, United States of America.

© Oxford University Press 2017

All rights reserved. No part of this publication may be reproduced, stored in
a retrieval system, or transmitted, in any form or by any means, without the
prior permission in writing of Oxford University Press, or as expressly permitted
by law, by license, or under terms agreed with the appropriate reproduction
rights organization. Inquiries concerning reproduction outside the scope of the
above should be sent to the Rights Department, Oxford University Press, at the
address above.

You must not circulate this work in any other form
and you must impose this same condition on any acquirer.

Library of Congress Cataloging-in-Publication Data
Names: Rosen, David H., 1945- author. | Hoang, Uyen B. (Uyen Bao), author. | Based on (work):
Reiser, David E., 1946- Medicine as a human experience.
Title: Patient-centered medicine : a human experience / David H. Rosen, Uyen B. Hoang.
Description: New York, NY : Oxford University Press, [2017] | Based on Medicine as a human experience /
David E. Reiser, David H. Rosen. c1984. | Includes bibliographical references.
Identifiers: LCCN 2016051453 | ISBN 9780190628871 (pbk.)
Subjects: | MESH: Patient-Centered Care—methods | Physician-Patient Relations | Health Communication |
Patients—psychology | Philosophy, Medical
Classification: LCC R726.5 | NLM W 84.7 | DDC 616.001/9—dc23 LC record available at
https://lccn.loc.gov/2016051453

This material is not intended to be, and should not be considered, a substitute for medical or other professional advice.
Treatment for the conditions described in this material is highly dependent on the individual circumstances. And, while
this material is designed to offer accurate information with respect to the subject matter covered and to be current as of
the time it was written, research and knowledge about medical and health issues is constantly evolving and dose schedules for medications are being revised continually, with new side effects recognized and accounted for regularly. Readers
must therefore always check the product information and clinical procedures with the most up-to-date published
product information and data sheets provided by the manufacturers and the most recent codes of conduct and safety
regulation. The publisher and the authors make no representations or warranties to readers, express or implied, as to the
accuracy or completeness of this material. Without limiting the foregoing, the publisher and the authors make no representations or warranties as to the accuracy or efficacy of the drug dosages mentioned in the material. The authors and
the publisher do not accept, and expressly disclaim, any responsibility for any liability, loss or risk that may be claimed
or incurred as a consequence of the use and/ or application of any of the contents of this material.

We owe special thanks to the following organizations and publishers:
1. The American Medical Association for permission to reproduce in the Foreword adapted excerpts from "The Physician as Communicator" by Norman Cousins, *Journal of the American Medical Association* 248: 587–589, 1982.
2. Belknap Press of Harvard University for poem number 1129 from *Poems of Emily Dickinson*, edited by Thomas H. Johnson, Cambridge, Mass., 1981.
3. Holt, Rinehart and Winston for "The Silken Tent" from The Poetry of Robert Frost, edited by Edward Connery Lathem, New York, 1967.
4. The American Psychiatric Association for "The Clinical Application of the Biopsychosocial Model" by George Engel, *American Journal of Psychiatry* 137: 535–544, 1980.
5. The Johns Hopkins University Press for "The Care of the Patient: Art or Science?" by George Engel, *Johns Hopkins Medical Journal* 140: 222–232, 1977.
6. The Williams and Wilkins Company for an excerpt from *Patient Interviewing: The Human Dimension* by David Reiser and Andrea Schroder, Baltimore, 1980.
7. Simon and Schuster for excerpts from *Heartsounds* by Martha Weinman Lear, New York, 1981.
8. The American College of Physicians for excerpts from "A Life Setting Conducive to Illness: The Giving-up/Given-up Complex" by George Engel, *Annals of Internal Medicine* 679, 293–300, 1968, and "Culture, Illness, and Care: Clinical Lessons from Anthropologic and Cross Cultural Research" by A. Kleinman, L. Eisenberg, and B. Good, *Annals of Internal Medicine* 88: 251–258, 1975.
9. Viking Penguin for an excerpt from *The Youngest Science* by Lewis Thomas, New York, 1983.
10. David McKay for "A Noiseless Patient Spider" from *Leaves of Grass* by Walt Whitman, Philadelphia, 1900.
11. St. Martin's Press for excerpts from *A Parting Gift* by Frances Sharkey, New York, 1982.

*This book is dedicated to our patients,
who have been our greatest teachers.*

# CONTENTS

Foreword by *Andrew Weil, MD*  ix
Foreword: Physician as Humanist by *Norman Cousins*  xi
Preface  xix
Prologue: An Early Career Female Physician's Perspective by *Uyen 3. Hoang*  xxi

1. Medicine as a Human Experience  1

2. Clinical Application of the Biopsychosocial Model  27
   *George L. Engel*

3. Care of the Patient: Art or Science?  43
   *George L. Engel*

4. The Doctor–Patient Relationship  53

5. The Patient-Centered Interview  69

6. The Experience of Illness and Hospitalization  87

7. The Nature of the Healing Process  107

Epilogue: Desiderata  139

Index  143

# FOREWORD

## By Andrew Weil, MD

When I was growing up in Philadelphia during the late 1940s and 1950s, our family doctor was a beloved general practitioner who made house calls, knew his patients well, worked hard, and was considered a friend. But, he wrote prescriptions in Latin to keep us in the dark about what they were, and we never questioned them or the treatments he ordered. He was the medical authority—a wise father figure; we were the children for whom he cared.

Medicine in mid-20th-century America was paternalistic and authoritarian, as it still is in many parts of Europe, Latin America, and Asia. But much has changed here in recent years. The Internet has leveled the playing field between doctors and patients, making medical knowledge available to all. The economic catastrophe that has engulfed our nation's healthcare system has weakened the authority of physicians. And the demand for "patient-centered medicine" has become a force to be reckoned with.

I teach and practice integrative medicine, which I believe must be the foundation of healthcare of the future. Integrative medicine insists that patients are not just physical bodies, but also they are mental/emotional beings, spiritual entities, and community members, and those other dimensions of human life must be taken into account to understand health and illness. The reigning biomedical model is obsolete. A new *biopsychosocialspiritual* model of medicine must supersede it. (*Integrative* is a more user-friendly term.)

Integrative medicine also emphasizes the importance of the practitioner–patient relationship in the healing process. Throughout history, in many diverse cultures, that relationship has been held special, even sacred. When a medically trained person sits with a patient and simply allows him or her to tell their story, that alone can initiate a healing response before any treatment is given. Sadly, today's corporatized healthcare does not allow for this. If medical visits are limited to 10 minutes or less, it is unlikely that a productive therapeutic relationship can form.

*Patient-Centered Medicine: A Human Experience* is a timely and welcome publication. Not only does it define the role of health professionals in the new model of medicine that is coming into being, it gives a great deal of practical advice about the attitudes and skills they should develop to care best for patients. Medical students and doctors in training will find it especially useful. I expect them, as physicians of the future, to lead the much-needed transformation of healthcare.

# FOREWORD: PHYSICIAN AS HUMANIST

*By Norman Cousins*

Written for the first edition of *Medicine as a Human Experience* by David E. Reiser and David H. Rosen

Drs. Reiser and Rosen have written a book filled with compassion and insight not only for patients but also for the singular and often complex young men and women who take upon themselves the healing role. I have been trying in recent years to find out as much as I could about the direction medicine seems to be taking. The authors provide some encouraging answers and point a path toward the resurrection of the principles of integration that are essential. By "integration" I am thinking not of a murky principle but of the need to affirm the importance of the human spirit, dignity, fullness, and hope in the philosophy of medicine.

Few things are more encouraging about modern medicine than the recognition that the psychological and the physiological are part of a totality; psychological and psychiatric problems are not merely aspects of medicine but are central to all medical practice. It is difficult to think of *any* relationship between a doctor and a patient that does not involve psychological and psychiatric competence by the physician. This is a fundamental issue.

Medical training tends to divide most subjects between "soft" and "hard." The hard subjects are defined as, or equated with, science: pathology, pharmacology, biochemistry, biophysics—everything that utilizes facts and numbers in one way or another. The soft subjects involve psychology, patient–doctor relationships, the philosophy of medicine, and the history of medicine.

When some subjects are defined as soft and others as hard, one makes value assignments. The hard is "good" and "dependable." The soft is "weak" and therefore to be disparaged. Yet 15 to 20 years after medical school, what happens? One discovers that the so-called, the supposed "hard" base of medicine breaks up—that the fact base of medicine is vulnerable. All one has to do is to look back over the past 25 years and certainly the past 50 years to see how much of medicine that was considered to be hard and indisputable has been refuted or replaced.

In many respects, the "soft" subjects have greater longevity. The way a doctor listens to a patient, his ability to inspire the patient's confidence, to communicate that which must be communicated in a way that does not destroy hope are things referred to as the "art of medicine." This is what medicine is all about, and this is what endures. As for science, certainly the scientific aspects of medicine are the foundation, but the "hard" facts keep changing because of the nature of both pure and applied research.

These matters Reiser and Rosen clearly grasp, and their book is an attempt to integrate "soft" and "hard," "science" and "art"—in short, to be truly scientific in the best sense of the term. Many textbooks have already been written that aspire to present students with a unifying view of patients and the practice of medicine. In this regard, *Medicine as a Human Experience* is not unique. What makes it unique, in my view, is the spirit its words embody, the attitude its pages communicate. The authors understand, and repeatedly demonstrate in this book, that the patient–physician relationship is a powerful, sometimes mysterious, frequently healing interaction *between human beings*. At the core of this interaction is communication.

Five years ago, I accepted an invitation to teach literature and philosophy to medical students at the University of California, Los Angeles, and to study problems in patient–physician relationships from the standpoint of patients. I also wanted to pursue research in a field of deep interest to me, the biochemistry of the emotions.

I thought I would have to brace myself for all the shocks that go with a new career, but I quickly discovered that physicians and writers have at least one thing in common: Communication is an important part of their trade. In journalism you live or die by your ability to use words. In health care the words a physician uses have a profound effect on the well-being of the patient. A doctor's words can be gate-openers or gate-slammers: They can open the way to recovery, or they can make a patient dependent, tremulous, fearful, resistant. The right words can potentiate a patient, mobilize the will to live, and set the stage for heroic response. The wrong words can produce despair and defeat or impair the usefulness of whatever treatment is prescribed. The wrong words can complicate the healing environment, which is no less central in the care of the patients than the factual knowledge that forms the basis of treatment.

Being able to diagnose correctly is one good test of medical competence. Being able to tell the patient what he or she has to know is another (and, as the authors later explain, both are essential skills of a "competent" physician). Now, I recognize the problems involved for the physician in proper communication. There is not only the problem of language itself—how to use words that do not confuse or mislead. There are also the professional problems—the obligation of the physician to inform the patient, the difficulties caused by the fact that patients vary in their ability to deal with the truth, the ease with which poor communication with the patient can spill over into tangled relationships and even malpractice suits.

Let me hover over some of these problems.

First of all, proper communication is one of the most difficult undertakings on earth. The older I get, the more I am forced to recognize that many or even most failures and break-downs have their origin in faulty communication. Whether we are talking the predicaments of human beings or the confrontations of nations, the inability of people to convey intention and meaning has been one of the prime causes of confusion and violence over the centuries. On a small but accessible level, you need go no further than the administration of hospital affairs to see how many errors, some of them serious, proceed out of faulty communications. Consider the wrong medications in the intravenous bottle, or the wrong pills, or the wrong quantities, or the hospital attendant who misinterprets instructions intended for one patient and applies them to another. Not infrequently, that attendant can fault ambiguous communications: the orders just were not clear enough.

Imprecision in communications, it goes without saying, is not confined to the medical profession. It is in the air. In the business world, blurred or faulty use of language represents the biggest single problem and single largest expense confronting any organization.

In my own contacts with patients, I have been made aware of the frequency with which they seem frightened or confused or immobilized as the result of their medical encounters. I allow for the possibility that their reactions may be the result of their own failures in understanding, but I am nevertheless struck with the fact that the relationship between patient and physician is often impaired because of sloppy communications.

Now we come to an entirely different problem. Even when the physician's message *is* clearly delivered and clearly understood, its effect may run counter to the well-being of the patient. Patients are not equally adept in their ability to handle the truth. Some may even be exposed to iatrogenic hazards if they are confronted at point-blank range with the fact of extreme illness.

One of the residents at UCLA spoke to me about a conference with a patient and the family, during which they were all expecting the attending doctor's verdict after a biopsy. The oncologist came in the room; the family was seated. He sat down, spread his hands, and said, "Well, I've got to let you have it." He said, "Your kidneys have crapped out." He said, "Your liver is crapped out. As a matter of fact, he said, "Everything is crapped out. That's the way it is." And he left.

Truth is the fashion these days. No one wants to stand against the truth. We all want the truth. But there are some problems here. The issue, it seems to me, is not do you tell the truth, but first do you really know the truth? Does any doctor really know enough to make a pronouncement of doom? Yes, he knows the basis of the evidence and on the basis of the averages that this patient may live just 3 or 4 months, but he is diagnosing an average—he is not really diagnosing a patient. No one knows enough about a human being to make a precise pronouncement of doom, and yet such pronouncements are made all the time. A good habit to get into is to ask yourself: Do you really know the truth in the first place?

Second, how do you deliver the truth? Do you deliver it as though you have a truckload of bricks to unload on a patient, or is a certain sensitivity called for? Do you deliver it in a way that crushes the patient's hope? Or could you find some way of allowing that patient to stay alive psychologically?

It may be said that the physician has no choice but to convey the facts flat out, that the danger of malpractice suits is such that the physician is forced to tell the patient the worst in unmistakable terms. At least, if the worst should happen, the physician cannot be accused of failing to prepare the patient—a failure for which he could be held legally accountable.

The essential question, perhaps, is whether the hard facts and nothing but the hard facts are always necessary or useful. Now, if the reason for the hard facts is the doctor's fear of legal reprisal, then we have to ask ourselves if there is a conflict of interests between the patient's need for treatment and the physician's need for legal protection. Consider the case of the San Francisco patient who had a biopsy of a lump in her breast and who telephoned the oncologist 3 days later asking about the result. She was told that such serious matters were never discussed over the telephone but that she would be informed in due course. She was. She was informed by *certified* letter. The letter was completely unambiguous. It said in the tersest language that she had a malignancy. There was certainly no failure here in communication, but there was certainly little regard for the effect that communication in this form would produce. With a registered receipt in his possession, the physician could protect himself against any possible accusation later that he had failed to make an accurate diagnosis. The woman was not so much told as notified, not so much instructed as sentenced.

Is it reasonable to ask if insensitive reference to the worst helps to bring on the worst? To what extent does the *unvarnished* recital of a negative prognosis have the effect of a hex? Physicians are obligated to use all the science at their command—chemotherapy, radiation, surgery—in an attempt to reverse or slow down a malignancy. For the same reason, the wise physician calls up his humanity to potentiate and motivate the patient. The mood and attitude of the physician as well as that of the patient are potent factors affecting treatment. For that reason alone, the physician should try to avoid a situation in which either one leaves an encounter in sheer terror and defeat.

In my current position, I have a chance to see patients at the request of doctors: patients who have given up and who need emotional support. The most difficult thing in dealing with these patients is not the illness but the psychology it engenders. Nothing is more inevitable in serious illness than the panic that accompanies it. Panic is the intense fire of disease. Panic is a disease by itself. Panic makes biochemical changes in the body. What happens when the doctor communicates with a patient in a way that intensifies that panic? Perhaps it might have been better in some instances not to have gone to the doctor at all.

The authors of this book draw for you a clear picture of the way panic and stress can throw the entire endocrine system into disarray. It is no accident that disease frequently and suddenly becomes intensified as the diagnosis is pronounced. The way a patient receives a diagnosis can have a profound effect on the course of the disease. This does not mean that the truth must be deferred or denied. It is a matter of attaching as much importance to the manner and style of communication as to any other aspect of medical care.

We are accustomed to thinking of iatrogenic problems in terms of the wrong medication, or mistaken surgery, or harm done in diagnostic procedures. But there are also psychological iatrogenic situations—what happens after a patient is sent into an emotional tailspin with physiological consequences as the result of the exchange with a physician?

Everything we have said so far points to this question: Is it possible to communicate negative information in a way that is received by the patient as a challenge rather than as a death sentence?

I believe it is. As the authors of this book repeatedly demonstrate, understanding how patients are affected by serious illness, as well as what illness they happen to have, paves the way for communicating without crippling.

Throughout the book, an attitude is evidenced that is conducive to treatment and recovery. The authors do not minimize the seriousness of a patient's condition. What they do, instead, is to put their emphasis on healing as a partnership. They describe what it is that modern medical science has to offer, what it is that the patient has to offer, and finally what the physician as a human being has to offer. They talk about the patient's resources and, equally important, about the resources of the healer.

We make a great mistake if we think that in a serious or terminal illness victory is represented only by some miracle that reverses the illness—some beautiful remission—and that defeat is represented only by death. An illness is similar to existence inside the concentration camps. There are many victories short of escape, many victories short of cure, and many defeats that are not marked by death. Even though we cannot expect ultimate victory, our existence is enriched or impoverished by the interim victories or failures within our reach.

A young boy says, "It was wonderful when mother opened her eyes and recognized me." Another patient is able to turn over in bed by himself, and yet another patient is able to hold out her hand. These are the moments that are made possible by the physician as humanist, the physician who does not equate healing with some rigid and narrow definition of biomedical cure, the physician who appreciates the importance in medicine of such imponderables as hope, dignity, courage, and yes, love.

I am reminded of one of the doctors at Encino Hospital, who had a judge as a patient. The judge was willing himself to die. The family was bereaved not just because of his impending death but because his character had changed so drastically under circumstances of extreme adversity.

The judge had always been a fighter, strong and resolute. Now he was giving up, and all he wanted to do was to die. His family hardly recognized him, but the doctor was wise enough to ponder, "You know, if we can just give this family one week—one week—with the judge as he used to be, not in terms of health, but in terms of the spirit as they have recognized it, it would make a very big difference to them for the rest of their lives.

The next day I was leaving for China, so at the doctor's request I went to the Encino Hospital that night. The judge—a tall man, six feet three inches—was wasting away. He was down to about 90 pounds. He could barely speak. He had been a reader of the *Saturday Review*, so there was some way for me to reach out to him and have him reach back.

He whispered. He spoke about the magazine and how he had read it all those years, and I said "Dr. Bluming asked me to come and see you because of the family."

He said, "What about the family?" in a high whisper; and I said, "Well, you know, cancer is the most contagious of diseases."

He said, "No, it's not."

I said, "Well, it is contagious in the sense that the grief is the virus, and sometimes the way we die helps to determine what happens to others; and when you look at the records, you find that wives follow husbands within a few months and husbands follow wives—and the inability to handle grief is really a virus."

"You know, your family has always seen you as a great fighter, and now you're going out of character."

He said, "I gotcha."

The next day, when I arrived in Hong Kong, I telephoned the Encino Hospital and talked with Dr. Bluming. He said, "Gosh! Something very strange and wonderful has happened. When they tried to hook the judge up to his intravenous this morning, he said, 'Turn the damn thing off and give me my breakfast the regular way.' I don't know how he got it down—but he did."

The doctor reported, "Two hours later, he asked his wife to come over to play a game of bridge. How they played that game of bridge. I'll never know." The next day, the judge even walked around the room.

When I got back 3 weeks later, I discovered that he had died just 2 days before my return. He not only lived out 1 week, he lived out three—and he did so with spirit. He found his victory, and the family found its victory, in an altered context that was real.

There are victories that are possible, and a physician is responsible for helping us to get the most out of whatever may be possible. In the final analysis, medicine is the science and the art of the possible.

As this volume makes clear, the doctor's job is not just to deal with the ultimates. The doctor's concern is with the intermediates that make up our day-to-day lives. Nothing is more wondrous than the ability of the human spirit to produce profound biochemical, physiological, attitudinal, and behavioral change, even though a cure is not possible. I have been mystified by this and at times ennobled. This, it seems to me, is the great experience within the reach of physicians. The present text offers a path toward that full realization.

Patients need and look for qualities in their doctors that go beyond technical competence. They want reassurance. They want to be looked *after,* not just looked *over.* They want to be listened to. They want to feel that it makes a difference to the physician, a very big difference, whether they live or die. They want to feel that they are in the doctor's thoughts. In short, patients are a vast collection of emotional needs. Yes, psychological counselors are very helpful in this connection, and so are the family and clergy; but the patient turns most of all and first of all to the physician. It is the physician's station that has most to offer in terms of those emotional needs. It is the person of the doctor and the presence of the doctor, just as much as—frequently more than—what the doctor does that create an environment for healing. The physician represents restoration. The physician holds the lifeline. The physician's words and not just his prescriptions are entwined in that lifeline.

This aspect of medicine has not changed in thousands of years. Not all the king's horses and all the king's men—not all the tomography and thallium scanners and two-D echograms and medicinal mood modifiers—can preempt the physician's primary role as the keeper of the keys to the body's own healing system. To the students who read, and more important *understand,* the spirit and the essence of this book, I would say, without hesitation or fear of hyperbole, you are medicine's future. You are also its only hope.

I pray that you will never allow your knowledge to get in the way of your relationship with your patients. I pray that all the technological marvels at your command will not prevent you from practicing medicine out of a little black bag if you have to. I pray that when you go into a patient's room you will recognize that the main distance is not from the door to the bed, but from the patient's eyes to your own—and that this distance is best traveled when the physician bends low to the patient's fear of loneliness and pain and the overwhelming sense of mortality that comes flooding up out of the unknown, and when the physician's hand on the patient's shoulder or arm is a shelter against darkness.

I pray that, even as you attach the highest value to your science, you will never forget that it works best when it serves your humanity. For, ultimately, it is our respect for the human soul that determines the worth of our science.

---

\* Norman Cousins was an American journalist, author, professor, and world peace advocate. He was editor of the *Saturday Review* magazine for many years.

# PREFACE

First of all we acknowledge the contributions of Drs. David Reiser and George Engel who, with David Rosen, published Medicine as a Human Experience in 1984. When planning to develop a revision of that work, however, we were unable to locate Dr. Reiser after an exhaustive search and Dr. Engel is deceased. As with the earlier book, this volume is written for all students in the healthcare professions, including but not limited to medicine, nursing, physical therapy, social work, occupational therapy, psychology, psychotherapy, counseling, and clergy. We deeply appreciate their creative ideas, compassion, empathy, social concern, and humanism. We hope it will help future healthcare providers to sustain and expand these attributes throughout their careers, so they may truly say their educational experiences have been meaningful, human ones. Beyond this, we hope this text is useful to all professionals involved in healing roles—in short, to everyone who truly cares for patients and their families. This is something that goes way beyond technical degrees.

This book evolved out of our teaching experiences both in medical schools and in our communities. Dr. Rosen founded, directed, and participated in the Psychiatric Aspects of Medical Practice, funded by the Kaiser Family Foundation at the University of California, San Francisco. Dr. Hoang, one of Dr. Rosen's former students, has always worked in community mental health. We both have a love of teaching students from the various healthcare areas. It is so important to assist students to remain self-aware and to use a scientific paradigm in clinical medicine based on George Engel's biopsychosocial model.

Both Drs. Rosen and Hoang are committed to helping students realize the importance of the doctor–patient relationship—in other words, the human dimensions of healthcare work. Like Dr. Reiser and the late Dr. Engel, we help students learn psychosocial skills, patient-centered interviewing, clinical reasoning, and knowledge essential for humanistic clinical work. It is our objective to provide a bridge between students' evolving knowledge and application of this knowledge to their work with patients and their families. We are both devoted to patient-centered interviewing, obtaining a complete history, and conducting an examination using a biopsychosocial approach. We realize this is a faculty/staff intensive, apprentice-based, clinical educational experience, but essential to all healthcare disciplines. We hope to aid all students in adapting to loss and life change, pregnancy and human sexuality, child and adolescent care, long-term care, psychopathology, and clinical reasoning using the biopsychosocial model.

We revised and updated this text because we believe students need a book that helps them make the transition from the classroom to working with patients easier and more meaningful. We provide general principles, illustrated clinically, designed to elucidate and enhance the practice of humane, empathic, patient-centered care in the clinical settings where students learn.

*Patient-Centered Medicine: A Human Experience* emphasizes the student healthcare professional's role in caring for patients as unique individuals, focusing on their psychological, philosophical, and social realities as well as their biological needs. Many students have expressed increasing concern over the trend toward fragmented, dehumanized healthcare. We share this concern, and this book is an attempt to address it. Throughout its pages, we convey the message that being knowledgeable about and sensitive to the human being on which we focus are the essential features of effective and successful care.

This volume concerns itself with caring for the whole patient, and outlines basic precepts involved in an empathic, biopsychosocial approach to healing. The prologue by Uyen Hoang is a practitioner's moving summation of her own experience working in the community—a piece that takes a candid look at traumas as well as triumphs. The first chapter outlines basic principles of medicine as a human experience and provides a template for the text. The next two chapters by George Engel concern the clinical application of the biopsychosocial model and the care of the patient. Chapter 4, "The Doctor–Patient Relationship," underscores the key nature of the human bond between the healthcare worker and the patient as partnership, which is essential to the healing process. Chapter 5 concerns itself with the patient-centered interview, a basic tool using the biopsychosocial approach. Chapter 6 focuses on the experience of illness and uses a developmental schema that highlights a patient's potential for growth, even while being sick. The last chapter, "The Nature of the Healing Process," emphasizes the known tangibles of scientific healthcare in the broadest sense that must be coupled with the intangibles of compassion, empathy, hope, and meaning if healing is to occur. In the epilogue, "Desiderata" guideposts are offered to help students find their way through the difficult maze we call education in the healthcare professions.

Didactic principles are always drawn from clinical experience, keeping the focus of the book where it should be—on the patient, a suffering fellow human being. We insist that patients be seen as people struggling with life and its often traumatic disruptions, never as interesting cases or examples of pathology.

We sense a change in healthcare education toward a more holistic paradigm. The challenge and responsibility for changing our healthcare professions rest with all of us. Fortunately, healthcare education has reviewed its educational goals and objectives to foster an understanding of healthcare as a personal human experience.

It is our hope that *Patient-Centered Medicine: A Human Experience* contributes in a small but meaningful way to making the practice of healthcare more comprehensive, more meaningful, more humane, and human. We intend this book to be a guide, a comfort, and an inspiration to young healthcare professionals as they pursue their own healing and the healing of their patients.

*David H. Rosen, MD*
Eugene, Oregon, USA

*Uyen B. Hoang, MD*
Auckland, New Zealand

# PROLOGUE: AN EARLY CAREER FEMALE PHYSICIAN'S PERSPECTIVE

*By Uyen B. Hoang, MD*

I was asked by my college mentor Dr. David Rosen to help update a text he had cowritten a little more than 30 years ago, a text he had gifted me for my college graduation long before I really knew medicine was my calling. What an honor! I was beside myself, wondering what meaningful ways I could contribute.

After rereading the text, I realized the gravity of the material laid out bravely years ago in an era dominated by the biomedical model of medicine—material that is equally relevant today, if not more, given the astonishing advances in science and technology amid the challenging demands of a complex healthcare system. Material that is timeless and actually required little updating. It is a privilege to have this opportunity to add to the discourse on a substantial topic in which Dr. David Rosen, Dr. David Reiser, and the late Dr. George Engel were ahead of their contemporaries in championing, when they all collaborated on the original text *Medicine as a Human Experience* (An Aspen Publication, 1984). The principles of what we today term as *patient-centered medicine* were discussed thoughtfully in the original text. My involvement serves to highlight why it has remained relevant (although self-evident) by providing a brief overview of milestones toward progressive reforms of the US healthcare system in parallel with medical and physician education reforms, and updating medical terminology and clinical examples, as applicable. I accepted this collaborative work as a sign of gratitude for my mentor, to share personal stories with the hope it may offer some comfort and pearls I wish I had known early on, and because I was in a creative space in which I found joy in writing.

Let me begin by providing a brief biographical sketch. I am a first-generation Vietnamese-born American raised in Texas, where I received my undergraduate and graduate medical education. After college, I joined a national teaching corp which led me to Los Angeles in 2001—a deeply riveting experience that shaped my trajectory in medicine. I returned to Texas in 2003 for medical school then relocated to Orange County, California, for residency in 2007. There, I trained as a psychiatrist across multiple settings, largely at the university medical center, community clinics, and a major health maintenance organization. My psychiatry education was balanced in psychopharmacology and psychotherapy, although it leaned toward a biological orientation. I worked with multidisciplinary teams and patients across varying models of care and diverse socioeconomic backgrounds, respectively. I remained in southern California for the early years of my practice postresidency before moving overseas—early years that were equally riveting in shaping the integrative psychiatrist I have become.

Psychiatry as I now practice in New Zealand has been transformative, in parallel with how my writing has evolved to transform me. My interest in writing actually grew from a personal quest to improve my clinical report as a means of communication. My writing matured as I advanced through the stages of physician training and as a result of being conscientious about my ability to communicate clearly to my patients and colleagues. It has become more streamlined, while managing the nuanced requirements from different services and health insurance providers.

During my formative years of residency training and beyond, I endeavored to provide a clinical report written in a way for readers to understand how I arrived at an impression and plan of care based on a cross-sectional assessment of the patient's presenting illness. I considered the context of antecedents against a background of data relevant to the patient's condition, which are standard to a comprehensive assessment (eg, past psychiatric history, risks when unwell, social history, physical health history, substance use, mental status examination). My clinical report was a tool to communicate information to providers involved in the patient's care. It was always written with the intention that, in my absence, another clinician unfamiliar with the patient could discern easily my rationale behind the current plan of care and how to proceed if providing coverage. Besides a means of communication, I also considered documentation from an indemnity perspective, as was emphasized during my training and reflected in the defensive style of practice around me. Considering it from my patients' perspective did not occur until later.

Four years after graduating from residency in 2011, I found myself in New Zealand simply in search of something greater. I was craving an intangible I could only describe as *expansion*. I viewed this time as a self-appointed sabbatical of sorts to gain experience for personal and professional enrichment. When David asked me to collaborate on this text in late 2015, I was in a space where I viewed my clinical writing in a different light. Layering on what I had learned in my training, there was a novel perspective I had never really considered before—a way to honor my patients' stories, written with sensitivity. A conversation with Dr. Debbie Antcliff, former Clinical Director of Community Mental Health Services under the Auckland District Health Board, would seed ideas for change. She challenged me gently to consider the clinical report from the patient's perspective, with respect to sensitivity toward the language of medicine. Questions I had not really considered before now arose. How would patients react to reading their story? How would it make them feel? Was there a message of hope I was holding for them when they could not go it alone? It was synchronicity in that this conversation with Debbie occurred at my friend Dr. David Kopacz's book reading of his important work, *Re-humanizing Medicine* (Ayni Books, 2014).

Dr. Antcliff's challenge resonated with me as I started to get my bearings as a consultant psychiatrist in Auckland at an inner-city community mental health center. What struck me early on were the daily morning team meetings during which my colleagues, a multidisciplinary team consisting of another psychiatrist, a registrar (resident equivalent in New Zealand), psychologists, and other health clinicians (social workers, nurses, and occupational therapists), were compelling storytellers who conveyed the life narratives of our patients in a light reflective of their complex tapestry. It captured their humanity without losing sight of germane data relevant to their presenting condition. It was a contrast to my style of systematic, technical reporting.

There was an implicit expectation for everyone to listen and give their undivided attention, in contrast to what I was accustomed to in similar team meetings in Orange County, during which the doctor was "listening" but reviewing charts and reports for the day simultaneously. In a similar vein, at a clinic in Riverside County, the doctor "listened" but intermittently stared at a screen and typed while interviewing, because this was the only way to see up to 18 patients a day, return phone calls and e-mails, renew prescriptions, complete requested forms, stay on track with key performance indicators, and finish in a Godly hour. I was that doctor. This was not how I trained nor how I desired to practice, but I simply had to adapt.

At a community clinic in Orange County, where the majority of patients were monolingual Vietnamese speakers, I mastered interviewing in Vietnamese while translating to English text as I typed at my computer. I adapted and, over time, developed an apologetic style asking for permission to continue in this way. As you can imagine, I had to make a concerted effort to stay attuned and be empathic under these conditions. It took immense mental effort—mental effort that eventually waned, unable to keep pace with competing demands.

Surprisingly, most of my patients did not mind because this was the healthcare system to which they had grown accustomed. I had developed a way to be efficient while being patient-centered (or so I thought), staying attuned to my patients and their values, not compromising the standard of care, *and* meeting workplace and health insurance demands. As best I could, I applied an integrative approach of using the biopsychosocial perspective in my practice, exploring spiritual and cultural identities when time permitted, and liaising with other providers as necessary. These tasks required an extraordinary amount of time outside what was allocated, and often meant working through lunch and staying late.

I was astutely aware of burnout; I experienced it throughout my teaching years (the main reason I left that profession), and intermittently in medical school and residency. Although this was a matter addressed at the residency level where I trained, it did not get the full attention it deserved, nor were there measures in place to monitor residents for burnout routinely, ironically in a profession of caring for others. As such, I was mindful of maintaining a healthy work–life balance, keeping a pulse on staying well, and, after training, continuing with individual psychotherapy for personal and professional support.

It was by design that I chose to be self-employed and had diversified my practice with organizations and programs with vision and leadership in which I believed and with clinical duties that seemed reasonable. So, it was easy to turn away group practices for which the expectation was 15- to 20-minute medication checks, and clinicians were incentivized by compensation (ie, the more patients you see, the greater the financial reward). Even with having to "adapt," this was not the care delivery model for me.

I opted for a mix of clinics where my appointments ranged from 40 to 90 minutes for new patients and 30 minutes for follow-ups. The volume of patients I saw in a day also varied depending on the clinic, averaging from 10 to 14 and peaking at 18. This seemed reasonable in the beginning, except for the occasional days at one clinic when I was expected to evaluate 3 new "straightforward" patients in a 2-hour block inclusive of time for documentation. To interview a "straightforward" new patient in 40 minutes meant sometimes skimming the surface and not delving into what makes them human. I adapted.

Despite the growing pains of starting out on my own and not having the safety net of an attending, it was quite exhilarating finally to have substantial earning power while doing work I found meaningful, after many long years slaving away as a trainee in debt. I maintained an average of 45 work hours weekly and would pick up extra weekend shifts periodically at two community clinics where my patients were predominantly Vietnamese with mixed levels of publicly funded health insurance—an underserved group that required being creative with limited resources.

At the peak of my earnings in Southern California, I was making 6 times my resident salary, which afforded a very comfortable lifestyle and the means to take unpaid leave for holiday and to fly home regularly to see my family in Texas. I was living the American dream, as the first to attend college in my family—a family that fled its homeland as refugees in search of opportunity and simply a better life for its children. I rose from humble beginnings to a privileged life in the service of others, with a sense of purpose to give back to communities where I began. What got in the way of my adapted practice of medicine? Burnout. And its insidious way of eroding one's spirit and will.

My wakeup call came in late 2012, when a patient delivered words no doctor wants to hear, "You lack compassion." At this time, I was scoring consistently above 90% in metrics for patient satisfaction, but this knowledge provided little comfort as my patient's experience confirmed what I had known. It was a message delivered in a measured way, prefaced by telling me he thought I was a skilled clinician/technician, but I lacked heart. The circumstances were complex because I had inherited both he and his wife as patients when I started work at this particular clinic. There was an obvious conflict of interest, which was unavoidable given clinic pressures. Although I had struggled at times to empathize with him during the course of treatment, I thought there was a reasonable degree of professional rapport to compensate. The awakening aspect came not only from the content of his message, but from my reaction (or lack of one).

On the surface, I managed this difficult situation to his satisfaction. He would be referred to another provider per his preference. As we ended that session, I listened respectfully, acknowledged his truth, and apologized for not providing the support he needed. It felt perfunctory. Inside I felt numb and disconnected. It was as if my empathy and compassion reserves were empty. You would expect such an admonishment to elicit a jarring effect. It did not have this effect immediately. In that moment, I was a shell of myself, unable to summon what gave me meaning in my work.

Principles and values that guided my way of being and how I practiced medicine, professional and personal supports, and robust self-care all failed to immunize me from burnout. I had thought naively that these measures would be enough, when, in fact, nothing would have been enough had I continued to "adapt" and permit conditions not conducive to my health nor that of my patients.

Weekly professional supervision helped me identify and accept what I was experiencing as burnout before it engulfed me completely. Although I had experienced varying degrees of it before and knew of its harmful effects, there was still shame attached to acknowledging burnout in myself. Perhaps this goes back to my days of teaching—a challenging period I have not fully unpacked. As an early career psychiatrist suffering from burnout, I was fortunate to have a close circle of female physician friends, and we spoke freely about our similar circumstances and their impact on our well-being. We all, ultimately, made changes in our practice to save ourselves.

The work of psychiatry (and doctoring) is immensely rewarding and demands a vital balance to self-sustain in a meaningful way—a vital balance to avoid burnout, that of emotional exhaustion, depersonalization, and a diminished sense of personal accomplishment.[1]

Even with improved workplace changes, the sequelae of burnout left me feeling diminished, which in turn sparked needed self-inquiry: questioning how I allowed myself to be so steeped in burnout before effecting change, questioning how I could expand on optimizing patient wellness beyond the standard of care as an American board-certified psychiatrist with a view for a greater integrative approach, questioning whether I would fully regain my spirit.

This self-inquiry led me to New Zealand in search of something greater, on a quest for expansion and truth. I came here with a finite time in mind: 1 year to explore and learn. I was surprised to find a practice that really suited me, a practice more amenable to fostering compassionate care. There are certainly clinical and systemic pressures with a growing population against limited resources for publicly funded national healthcare. Although, compared with how I practiced before, these conditions overall permit greater space for a compassionate practice that leaves me less vulnerable to burnout. There is more emphasis on a work–life balance here with respect to annual leave, sick leave, and continuing professional education leave (which is inclusive of self-development practices such as yoga and meditation). I work at a clinic where the morale is strong and there is a genuine sense of caring among colleagues. When I suddenly lost a patient (accidental death vs suicide), there was permission to grieve openly, to take the day off from clinical duties, and to process in a proper debriefing—simply, all-around support. I see fewer patients in a day, and am able to provide integrative care without stretching myself like I did before. I am surrounded by seasoned clinicians—in particular, master class-level psychologists to whom community patients have access. There is greater collaboration and a shared sense of responsibility—a different hierarchy in which everyone's input is valued and brings value with it. A major aspect of medicine is about building and maintaining relationships, and I have learned a great deal in observing the different styles of how others achieve this here.

In hindsight, what I learned is the importance of recognizing when change is necessary, when certain conditions no longer permit wellness and quality, safe practice. I hope to recognize early signs of burnout when it recurs (the work of caring for others makes me vulnerable) and to have the capacity to summon courage and wisdom to effect change, however small or grand. I have been fortunate to have the freedom to take such a leap in my move to New Zealand, without having to consider Whanau[2] responsibilities. When my initial year-long commitment came to an end, I happily accepted an offer for a permanent position to continue to explore the reasons that brought me here.

With respect to personal development, I have found a mindfulness practice that resonates and keeps me grounded, and from which I have noted enduring positive effects as I continue to deepen my practice. Encouraging my patients to explore mindfulness now has more meaning when I can share my personal experience. With respect to professional development, I had hoped to be enlightened by novel healing and recovery methods; instead, I found myself humbled, admiring in my new colleagues the mastery of essential skills: that of listening, validating, storytelling, and sharing risks and holding hope collectively. I felt like I was beginning again, armed with renewed interest and optimism in doctoring.

Collaborating on this book has been a needed refresher and has enhanced my practice of psychiatry, of patient-centered medicine. Reviewing the original material has been timely and impactful, returning me to the basics that have immeasurable therapeutic effects, such as that of simply listening.

Seated with my Kiwi[3] colleagues for our morning team meeting, I began to listen again with an ear for details of a different sort—what I had enjoyed before when I was unencumbered by metrics, checklists, and competing demands. It was not an adapted way of "listening," that of distilling a patient's story down to target symptoms and differential diagnoses, it was listening for what gives them meaning, joy, and hope—what defines their humanity. This experience abroad has been an opening to appreciate again what had been at times forgotten in the grind of psychiatry as I had practiced before. It has given me pause to acknowledge the immense privilege I have as a physician, as a caregiver, as a healer.

## REFERENCES

1. Maslach C, Jackson SE, Leiter MP. *The Maslach Burnout Inventory*. 3rd ed. Palo Alto, CA: Consulting Psychologists Press; 1996, 2010. All versions of this document, and the manual, are now available at Mind Garden. http://www.mindgarden.com/117-maslach-burnout-inventory. Accessed September 7, 2016.
2. Whānau is a Maori concept of family, close-knit friendships, and community. On a deeper level, it encompasses physical, emotional, and spiritual dimensions. The Maoris are the indigenous population of New Zealand. Walker T. *Whānau – Māori and family – Contemporary understandings of whānau, Te Ara – the Encyclopedia of New Zealand*. 2011. http://www.TeAra.govt.nz/en/whanau-maori-and-family/page-1. Accessed September 7, 2016.
3. Kiwi is a colloquial term used to describe New Zealanders. Phillips J. *Kiwi, Te Ara - the Encyclopedia of New Zealand*. 2007; 2010. http://www.TeAra.govt.nz/en/kiwi. Accessed September 7, 2016.

# 1

## MEDICINE AS A HUMAN EXPERIENCE

We had just finished bedside rounds during which we interviewed a dying man. The interview had been sensitive. Subsequent discussion was lively but thoughtful. We asked why this suffering man felt compelled to deny how sick he was. The group felt animated and engrossed. Soon the students began linking events from the man's childhood to his coping style in the present. The connections seemed to make sense and helped us all to understand the patient better.

Then Jeff, a bright but skeptical student, pursed his lips.

"Okay," he said. "I buy it. Losing his father as a kid does relate to the way he is coping now. And I feel I understand him better as a person, which is good .... But so what?"

Silence.

"Really," Jeff persisted. I'm not putting this stuff down. I agree it's nice to understand our patients and that often doctors don't. But I still say—so what? What can I do practically? Now that I know all this, how do I help him?"

Jeff was not being simple-minded, prejudiced, or oppositional. He really did not understand what we ourselves had come to take so unquestioningly for granted—that empathy, understanding, and insight do help our patients, often help them a lot. At that moment, we also realized something else. The failure to comprehend lay less with Jeff than with ourselves. Despite the best intentions, we had still failed to make it clear to Jeff why understanding patients is not simply "nice" and "interesting" but absolutely essential to good medical care. Moreover, we must finally confess, the explanation that Jeff needed and deserved turned out not to be so simple to deliver.

On the other hand, the answer to Jeff's question—but put in reverse—is no more simple. The question is: Why is the importance of understanding the whole person, and not just fragments of him, so widely ignored and denigrated in modern medicine? How could this not be clear? How could it happen that Jeff's medical education would leave him bewildered about such fundamental truths instead of enlightened and reassured?

It is not our intent, however, to answer these questions, though they do cry out for answering. Rather, we will attempt to respond to the question Jeff asked, for it is a pivotally important one. Is the concept of medicine as a human experience really practical? Does it, in fact, make a difference with patients in the office and at the bedside? In short, is it merely "nice"—or does it help?

The opening passage of the original manuscript, *Medicine as a Human Experience* by David E. Reiser and David H. Rosen[1] is as relevant today as it was more than 3 decades ago. The clinical example just presented inspired much of the original manuscript, and guides our revision as we attempt to respond to the question Jeff asked, for—as mentioned—it is a pivotally important one. Is the concept of medicine as a human experience really practical?

A historical perspective is revealing. Clearly, the plea for empathic physicians is not, in itself, new. It is at least as old as medicine and as new as this text. The idea has had impassioned and articulate proponents all along. From this, we must infer the champions of empathy down through the decades also encountered resistance and perplexity from colleagues and students who were just as incredulous as Jeff. Conceptually, this is important, for it means that contemporary medical education is not wholly to blame for the problem. Medicine is currently fraught with serious shortcomings as medical science and technology continue to advance in an increasingly complex healthcare system. However, too many of its critics assume, naively and incorrectly, that dehumanization and lack of true holism in medicine are relatively new and therefore exclusively the fault of science and high technology.

The problem is not new. If it were, the Father of Modern Medicine, William Osler, would not have been pleading the same case with his colleagues more than a century ago, and Hippocrates long before that. All along, at least some physicians seem to have been saying rather skeptically, as Jeff did, "Okay, but so what?"

During the 32 years since the publication of Reiser's and Rosen's original work, have medical and physician education reforms progressed to a point where we no longer need to advocate for humanistic care as encapsulated in the patient-centered model? If inclusive in the curriculum, is it embedded and deserving of equal attention to its biomedical counterpart? If mastery of this humanistic dimension of medicine is achieved, is it then immune from the ailments of a healthcare delivery system that can both uplift as well as erode? These were questions that arose during the work of revising the original text.

Let us review a number of milestones throughout the course of healthcare, medical, and physician education reform. In 1999, the Institute of Medicine (IOM) released *To Err Is Human: Building a Safer Health* System,[2] in which it referenced the Quality of Health Care in America Committee of the IOM as concluding, "it is not acceptable for patients to be harmed by the health care system that is supposed to offer healing and comfort—a system that promises *First, do no harm*" (p. 2). The crisis of patient safety resulting from medical errors in the United States could no longer be ignored. Medical errors were said to arise from a faulty system, processes, and conditions, which led to mistakes and failure to prevent harm. In 2001, the Quality of Health Care in America Committee of the IOM followed up with *Crossing the Quality Chasm: A New Health System for the 21st Century*,[3] which called for a "fundamental, sweeping redesign of the entire health system," not merely "incremental improvements in current systems of care" (pp. 2, 2). The IOM called for all healthcare constituencies to adopt a shared, strategic vision for improvement in delivering high-quality healthcare. There were 6 specific aims[3,4] for healthcare to be: safe, effective, timely, equitable, efficient, and *patient-centered*. In 2003, the Committee on the Health Professions Education Summit Board on Health Care Services of the IOM released *Health Professions Education: A Bridge to Quality*,[5] which was informed by ideas developed from an interdisciplinary summit on educational reforms—namely, how to integrate a core set of 6 competencies, which included *patient-centered care*.

The Institute of Medicine defines *patient-centered care*[3-5] as: "Providing care that is respectful of and responsive to individual patient preferences, needs, and values, and ensuring that patient values guide all clinical decisions". For patient-centered care to be effective, it must be delivered in the context of a collaborative, shared decision-making process. Patient-centered care does not undermine the doctor's weighted role in helping patients make an informed decision that aligns with their values and clinical needs on balance with standard of care guidelines.

Around the same time the IOM's staggering reports drew tremendous public attention about the state of our healthcare system, in 1999 the Accreditation Council for Graduate Medical Education (ACGME) launched a long-term initiative—the Outcomes Project[6-8]—prompting widespread, fundamental changes in physician education: a paradigm shift from the traditional structure and process-based structure to a competency-based framework. The American Board of Medical Specialties and the ACGME endorsed 6 general competencies for graduate medical education[6,7]: patient care, medical knowledge, practice-based learning and improvement, interpersonal and communication skills, professionalism, and systems-based practice. This new framework served to set clear and high standards for essential dimensions required of physicians to provide quality patient care and to work effectively in an evolving, healthcare delivery system. The next phase established *milestones*[9] to operationalize the competencies to meaningful educational and clinical outcomes at the level of the individual learner and the residency program. Subsequent phases were said to move gradually toward integrating the competencies fully with learning and clinical care, then toward developing models of excellence—a work that remains in progress at the updating of this text. The mastery of these competencies speaks to achieving humanism in medicine as guided by the patient-centered care approach, which is evident later when we discuss the foundational principles.

In 2009, the ACGME held a design conference to explore how principles of patient-centered care (and family-centered care) can be implemented in settings where residents learn and participate in care.[10] Across diverse programs represented, there was a lack of uniformity on how this aspect of education was prioritized, and it was not uncommon for it to be on the lower end. Barriers and strategies were identified in achieving this competency, and the overarching consensus for this type of care to be sustainable was it required a "fundamental expectation for resident learning and attainment of competence.[10]"

In 2014, the IOM released a report titled *Graduate Medical Education That Meets the Nation's Health Needs*,[11] which focused on the extent to which the current system supports or creates barriers to producing a physician workforce ready to provide high quality, *patient-centered*, and affordable health care. That same year, the Association of American Medical Colleges released its *Optimizing: A Five-Year Road Map for America's Medical Schools, Teaching Hospitals, and Health Systems*[12] to optimize graduate medical education in which it proclaimed the "imperative for physicians to be compassionate champions for health has never been stronger" (p.5).

Only in April 2015 did the Medical College Admissions Test (MCAT) undergo a major and needed revision since its inception in 1928, prompted by two expert panel reports on competency-based medical education.[13] The new MCAT revision reflected an assessment of competencies expected of entering medical students per the Admission Initiative of the Association of American Medical Colleges.[14] For the first time, the MCAT included social and behavioral sciences content. The MCAT revision sought to acknowledge the importance of the biopsychosocial model of health, as evidenced by the new foundational concepts. The Psychological, Social, and Biological Foundations of Behavior comprised 5 (half!) of the 10 Foundational Concepts. The biopsychosocial model, which we explore later in depth, seeks to understand the patient's experience of illness holistically, and thus inform a patient-centered care approach. For completeness, the remaining 5 foundational concepts include Biological and Biochemical Foundations of Living Systems (3) and Chemical and Physical Foundations of Biological Systems (2).

Institutional and systematic translational change from the national level to programs to individual learners can move at a glacial pace, so it is incumbent upon our future doctors to seek out resources to enhance their learning. These educational benchmarks make a compelling case that the patient-centered approach is in its early phase of integration into learning and clinical care. It deserves the full attention of not only medical students and residents, but also, perhaps, of early to late career physicians. For students and residents, we hope this text serves as an adjunct to this effect. For those in practice who may feel diminished given the pressures of our current system, we hope this text refreshes and reminds you why you chose this noble and meaningful profession.

Our purpose in this chapter and throughout the rest of this book is to examine the principles that underlie the foundation of patient-centered care, a shift from the historical paradigm in medicine, which was in favor of the illness and doctor-centered approach. Major contributors to the patient-centered framework[15,16] acknowledge the biopsychosocial perspective in conceptualizing and implementing patient-centered care. The next two chapters are unedited contributions by the late George Engel from the original manuscript, and serve to contrast these differing views and describe the conception of the biopsychosocial model.

We address the essence of Jeff's question—the "so what?" part—by delineating what we believe to be four essential principles that underlie all of medicine as a human experience. They are *acceptance, empathy, conceptualization*, and *competence*. We believe these four elements comprise the foundation of *patient-centered medicine;* requisite in preparing physicians for the 21st century and beyond, as "compassionate champions for health." And we hope to make clear this is where the most effective, most human kind of medicine should always be centered. In elaborating on each of these principles, we try especially to make a case for their practical importance—why they are therapeutic, indeed essential, to our patients' welfare. Essential, not just "nice."

# THE FOUR PRINCIPLES OF MEDICINE AS A HUMAN EXPERIENCE

## Acceptance

At a conference on healing, Dr. Stephen Ray, an unusually sensitive, open physician who practiced plastic surgery at the University of Rochester, expressed his feelings about working with the severely deformed:

> Before I enter the room to see such a person, I clear my mind of prejudices and preconceptions. I remind myself that all of nature is part of some universal order and is therefore harmonious and beautiful. Then, if I walk into the room and see a man or woman whose face has been scarred beyond recognition, I do not see the grotesqueness but find myself thinking of spiritual things—ancient craggy rock faces, gnarled old trees. It's odd—but with this attitude, where others find ugliness, I can discern beauty.

What Dr. Ray is displaying is acceptance, a trait we believe is fundamental to all truly effective patient care. It is important to be clear what we mean by this simple word. Certainly *acceptance* has many commonplace meanings: acceptance of responsibility; acceptance of obligation; acceptance of assignments, tasks, and deadlines. Of course, we mean all of these, but we also mean something much more specific, more basic to the warp and weft of medicine itself. In its most fundamental sense, acceptance means the doctor takes the patient—the person as he is—into her mind, her heart, and her conscience. It is not an action, but an encompassing attitude. Furthermore, this attitude is not "mystical." Rather, it is embedded in what is most phylogenetically and ontogenetically basic to the human being. The doctor who fails to perceive this will never understand the essence of patient care and healing.

To develop this line of reasoning, permit us two excursions from what one normally thinks of as being a part of medicine. The first excursion is into etymology, the origins of our symbols and the conceptions of ourselves that are embedded in our language: *Accept* comes from the Latin verb *accipere*. It means "to take or receive." The word in turn is derived from a preposition, *ad* (meaning "toward") and *capere* (meaning "to take"). Note how similar *capere* is to two closely related Latin words: *caput* and *cephalicus*. Both of these words mean "the head." The origins of our language most likely reflect an innate appreciation that acceptance, on its deepest level, is mental, not physical. We embrace people most intimately not with our arms, but with our minds, and with that universal metaphor for mind, our hearts. Thus the fourth listed definition of "accept" in Webster's Third International Dictionary is just this—"to receive into the mind."

Why is this concept important? What does it have to do with modern medicine? The answer, we believe, lies in its intrinsic emphasis on receptivity rather than on action. Progressively, medicine (and indeed technological society itself) has grown more action oriented, yet acceptance reminds us that, at the deepest level, humans need to be received, embraced, taken in, incorporated—all far more quiet and receptive modes of relatedness than those to which we are usually accustomed.

A key line of evidence for the importance of acceptance in medicine as a human experience is found in the phenomenon of human bonding. Multiple studies have made abundantly clear, maternal acceptance is no mere nicety. Along with food and warmth, maternal acceptance is essential for normal human development. Observe a mother with her young infant—a 3-month-old, for example. She holds the infant to her breast, almost always with its head on the left, over her heart. She gazes into its eyes, and the child gazes back. Vocalizations are minimal and those present consist of sights, soft whispers, and coos. There is little motor activity. The mother's expression is serene. The baby's body tone is relaxed. If the baby is breastfeeding, its hand may reach out and gently stroke the mother's breast, or perhaps explore the contours of her mouth or hair. The mother, in turn, strokes the baby gently and coos. It is a moving and beautiful sight. It is also the biology of survival.

Now observe the child when it is not being held or, equally distressing for the infant, being held improperly, unempathically by a tense, distracted, or indifferent mother. It may begin to cry and scream. Its body tonus becomes tense, its back and neck arch. When such distress occurs in a well-nurtured baby, the mother who is sensitive to her child responds quickly, knowing "instinctively" what her child needs—more milk, a dry diaper, a good burping, to be warm, to be held.

We are all moved by such a sight. It is lovely. However, such a response, unamplified by a scientific understanding of what is actually transpiring in the dyad, misses the fundamental point: We are witnessing here a basic biological process, one essential to the survival of the species. This early trust contains the origins of later forms of human acceptance—embracing, receiving, taking into the mind. Note especially what is *not* present. The baby's motor activity is greatly reduced. His vocalization and the mother's are minimal and muted in tone. Silence, touch, and eye contact predominate. In fact, an increase in vocalization and motor activity usually signals increased infantile tension and distress. The entire sequence occurs with a minimum of action, conscious thought, or words. We see the absence of this process at times when the mother is having difficulty with her child or is unavailable emotionally. Such mothers typically talk a lot and move a lot, alternating between detachment and activity. Their voices are loud. They may tickle the baby, say "There, there!" loudly, and shift the baby from shoulder to shoulder. As the mother's frustrated activity increases, the infant in turn becomes progressively more distressed, vocal, and hyperactive. What does this have to do with understanding patients? The answer is: a great deal!

In a similar vein, the Still Face Experiment by Dr. Edward Tronick and colleagues in 1975[17] described a phenomenon of social reciprocity between infant and mother, how an infant reacts after a few minutes of repeated attempts to engage a nonresponsive, expressionless mother back to the usual reciprocal pattern. Subsequent to failed attempts, the infant withdraws. When the mother resumes back to normal relating, the infant reciprocates equally, engaging warmly again with the mother. The still face effect is also elicited by fathers, strangers, and even by televised images of adults. It remains one of the most replicated findings in developmental psychology.[18]

Let us go back to the healthy, secure baby. Time passes and, with trust and acceptance as building blocks, the infant grows. Cognition increases and his world expands. He gains motor control and explores his environment. Soon he develops language and, with language, the capacity for abstraction—words, actions, ideas, and purposes. During adulthood, only the most intimate and special of circumstances, such as sexual intimacy, permit the typical grownup to let go and revert to that earlier state of tension release and nonverbal bliss. It is this capacity to surrender willingly to the care of another, to let go of one's customary and excessive self-control, that many adults find so exceedingly difficult. Commonly, we say, "I just can't relax." Often we really mean, "I can't entrust myself totally to another."

Consider now the plight of our patients. When a person is very sick, in pain, in a hospital, nature has potentially played a cruel trick on him indeed. Although he is not a baby, he is at risk of becoming or being as helpless as a baby. He is dependent, passive, and frightened, sometimes terribly afraid to move. Once again, he is dependent on caretakers. For the first time since he was a tiny baby, feeding and bowel care are again in the hands of others. The nature of severe illness itself triggers a regression to such a state of dependency (so similar to infancy). Patients fight it in different ways, but the regression itself is usually inevitable. We see the most extreme example of it in the total passivity and helplessness of the patient who has given up, but lesser degrees abound. Many patients fight the dependency very hard. Cassem and Hackett[19,20] suggest, however, that patients who can accept this inevitable regression and allow themselves to become dependent and place total, even idealized faith in their doctors may sometimes be better off. The patients who fight their dependency, on the other hand, may tend to encounter more problems. Perhaps this is why doctors are such notoriously poor patients. As a rule, physicians are reluctant to relinquish control, even when it would be entirely appropriate to do so.

Here we have it then: a patient who is disorganized, suffering, and regressed, but usually hating the regression itself and fighting it actively. Enter the doctor—a person who, for many reasons, may be especially afraid of such disorganization and helplessness in himself. Typically, we doctors tend to talk a lot. From the outset, our questions are very focused, content oriented, and paced in rapid, staccato succession. We issue instructions. We move constantly, fidgeting and probing, fingering our reflex hammers and stethoscopes. Too often, the result is a patient who does not feel accepted. Akin to the agitated baby in an anxious mother's arms, the jostling and shaking that characterizes too many physicians' styles increases the patient's fearfulness and tension. This is why doctors need to learn attentiveness, receptivity, openness, increased tolerance of feelings, and silence, so the patient can begin to relax, feel protected, and begin to trust. Such acceptance is an ingredient of healing—one that goes far beyond any mere polishing of bedside manner. It is an essential response to yearnings locked deep in all human beings. Effective doctors must learn to resonate with this basic longing and give over and submit to trust in their patients.

Consider again how this basic, evolutionary need is expressed in our language. Listen to how we speak of "good doctors." We say they are *compassionate, warm, feeling,* and possessing a big *heart.* When patients feel understood by such a doctor, they state frequently that "the doctor accepted me," and the patient is *touched* by such acceptance—"I can trust her." As you listen to these phrases, consider their physicality, think back to that baby once again held in his mother's arms, warm and safe, head against the breast, listening to the rhythmic pounding of the heart. The doctor–patient relationship is rooted in biology and evolution, not in mysticism or mere sentiment.

To accept the patient, we must learn to listen better. We must learn to permit feelings to emerge more. We must become more receptive. We need to master the difficult act of being quiet. Although this aspect of healing has been woefully neglected, scientific exploration in this area is both important and possible, just as it has proved to be in the study of the infant–mother dyad, another subject originally relegated to sentiment and mystery. The clue to many illnesses may lie in the physiological response of a distressed organism when it needs soothing, comfort, and quiet nurturance. Just as was true for the infant, the *lack* of these responses (internally or from the environment) could, conceivably, lead to altered physiological states predisposing to disease. Identifying such phenomena would obviously be important in understanding illness onset. Similarly, learning how to soothe may be a neglected yet critical aspect of healing required even after the disease has been cured.

Whether through ignorance or for other reasons, modern medicine too often seems to have lost sight of these human requirements. Instead of listening, we talk. Instead of accepting patients, we subject them to tests and procedures. In place of a gentle touch, we also offer a pill. We have lost sight of too much that is essential to healing, including the importance of acceptance.

## Empathy

Empathy is the second principle of patient-centered medicine. Its importance has been widely stressed along with its dimensions, described by many writers concerned with the doctor–patient relationship. It has been defined variously, with most of the definitions attempting to connote an emotional stance that avoids extremes of overidentification on the one hand and excessive emotional detachment on the other. A useful definition describes empathy as the ability to understand and share in another's feelings fully, coupled with the ability to know those feelings are not identical to one's own.

Defining empathy may be difficult, but achieving it is even harder. Most students find that they tend to oscillate between periods of overidentification with patients and periods of excessive detachment. The notion of striking a balance is obviously appealing but not simple to effect. In truth, accurate and consistent empathy with patients is an exacting skill—one that requires years of experience and effort to develop fully.

For the student who is first approaching the task, it is important to understand empathy's dynamic quality. It is a fluid process, not some ideal fixed point between "too close" and "too far." It is useful to think of the empathic process as analogous to multiple frames in a motion picture. Although the movie one sees on the screen seems smooth and consistent, slowing down the frames reveals rapid and remarkable shifts. Imagine that observing empathy is a bit like observing a film of a hummingbird, apparently poised in one spot. If we slow down the action and study each frame, we would see thousands of small corrections, constant shifts and changes in the yaw and pitch of the bird's beating wings. Analogously, a doctor does not really stay poised at some ideal distance from a patient to empathize, although it might appear so. Actually, with a speed and fluidity that does indeed resemble the beating of a hummingbird's wings, an empathic physician moves about constantly—extremely close to a patient one minute, more detached the next, somewhere in between these extremes most of the time. To illustrate this process more clearly, we turn our focus to two hypothetical cases. For didactic purposes, let us indulge in the luxury of modern cinematography: stop-action, slow motion, and instant replay.

The first case is a relatively simple one. We need only observe it in slow motion. Imagine a doctor is interviewing a young woman in her 20s who has been hospitalized for a flare-up of diabetes that worsened after her mother died the month before. The patient's lips begin to quiver and tears well up in her eyes. The doctor, in turn, feels himself growing teary-eyed and fears momentarily that he, too, will burst into tears. He draws back and regards his patient for a moment from a safer distance. Quickly, regaining his composure, he almost instantaneously draws closer again and says softly, "You still miss her terribly, don't you?" The patient now sobs openly. The net effect of the interaction could be described as "empathic," but the actual process was far more fluid and dynamic.

Physicians who have achieved empathy possess a very potent tool. First, they can articulate for their patients what they are actually experiencing, which can be highly therapeutic in its own right. Perhaps more important, accurate empathy enables physicians to avoid many of the communication breakdowns, frustrations, and hostilities that arise so often in clinical work. In our experiences, the vast majority of these disruptions begin with a breakdown in empathy. This is relevant in today's climate of medical education in which a significant decline in empathy occurs during the third year of medical school—time when empathy is most essential, given the shift toward patient care activities.[21] This breakdown in empathy includes its erosion early in training when empathy is not grasped accurately.

The usefulness of accurate empathy goes further. As everyone knows, doctors do not treat patients in a vacuum. Patient care occurs in a complex social system—typically during the student's clinical years in a hospital ward. The tensions, hostilities, counterhostilities, flirtations, and minor irritants that so frequently spring up in these settings can bewilder physicians and hurt patient care. Such occurrences are common, perhaps, but we believe they warrant a closer look. Again, let us turn on our magic camera and view another hypothetical case. This one turns out to be more complex and unsettling.

Michael Smith is a youthful-looking junior student doing his first rotation on Internal Medicine. The setting is a crowded, hectic ward in a county hospital. Michael's patient is a 47-year-old unemployed "waitress" named Johnnie. In fact, Johnnie is a sex worker who has an alcohol use disorder. She is in a troubled relationship with a partner, who is her pimp, and has been in prison several times. Currently, she is in the hospital for severe abdominal pain, possibly alcohol-induced pancreatitis.

A hard-edged, boisterous woman, she seems to get along well enough with the resident and intern who are taking care of her. Their interactions at the bedside seem amiable enough, filled with gruff joking and double entendres. However, this apparent ease of rapport is not destined to be for Michael. We pan in on the action as he approaches her bedside, just after the intern and resident have left. Michael has been assigned to do her admission history and physical. The resident told him earlier, snidely and barely out of the patient's earshot, "Have we got a good one for you."

From the outset, Michael senses Johnnie absolutely hates him. To illustrate what soon transpires, we stop the action at several points and see what is going on in the individual frames.

Initially, Michael fidgets nervously, the back of his neck heating up, as Johnnie beholds him with a silent but scornful scowl. He fumbles as he tries to get his ophthalmoscope set up.

Suddenly, Johnnie crows out, "How old are you anyway?"

"Twenty-three," Michael mumbles uncomfortably.

"Why the hell are they sending in a scrub?!" she retorts. "Am I suppose to be your guinea pig?"

Michael squirms and mumbles something.

"I don't like your attitude," she says snidely. "I may be a county patient, but I'm no fool. Go get one of the *real* doctors to examine me!"

Mike withers inside, his palms now perspiring profusely. He trembles with humiliation and anger.

Let's stop the action and observe what is happening.

Clearly, Johnnie has seen right through Michael's insecurities, attacking him precisely where he is most vulnerable—his concerns about his youth, inexperience, and ineptitude.

Let the camera roll again. Initially, Michael tries to handle the problem by being polite and conciliatory, but it does not work.

"I'm not your guinea pig!" Johnnie snaps. "Don't come near me!"

At this point, Michael decides to sound more "authoritative," as he imagines his resident would in this situation.

"Listen, Ms. Johnson!" he says in his gruffest voice. "I am here to examine you. This isn't a private hospital. This is important! There are other patients waiting, so we need to get this done now."

Pause the action.

Michael has now puffed up his chest and tried to seem as stern and "physicianly" as he can. He hopes this will force his rambunctious patient to comply, but it is not to be.

Roll the camera. Johnnie now squints at Michael with sardonic amusement. A wry smile then breaks through the leathery dissipation of her worn face. With slow and deliberate measure, she says, "Back off! Come near me and you'll see." She grabs her IV pole, which begins to totter dangerously. "Don't test me! Scram or I'm gonna smash this upside your head!"

Cut!

What has happened? For very understandable reasons, Michael has not been able to empathize. This is hardly surprising, and Johnnie is no gem, but such an explanation does not suffice. To begin with, Michael is already self-conscious about his inadequacies. Confronted with this difficult, belligerent patient, his composure evaporates quickly. He then tries to act tough, but to no avail. Moreover, from the looks of the saline bag tottering menacingly on its pole, he is in some danger of getting clobbered.

What went wrong? Essentially both parties were too wrapped up in themselves to have empathy for the other. It is hard to know precisely what was on Johnnie's mind; she probably was angry about being objectified by the house officers, enraged yet intimidated. So, she took out her fury on the inexperienced, vulnerable medical student, Michael. Michael, too, had entered the interaction already distracted, preoccupied with his own feelings of inadequacy. As soon as she shot off her "zinger," Michael reacted as though the attack were all too real. We repeat: *as though it were real*. Michael, as is so typical of doctors, then responded to Johnnie in suit. Assuming her accusation had legitimacy, he felt he had no option except to refute her logic. As doctors often do, he tried, initially, to be conciliatory and play nice. When that failed, he tried to pull rank. Essentially, however, he responded to her accusation at face value and attempted to restore his position by proving her wrong.

Because this is a hypothetical situation, we can indulge in the luxury of an instant replay. Let us imagine that Michael seeks the counsel of an attending physician whom he respects and trusts. Let us be a little frivolous and imagine the attending right there in the hospital, although it is 11:00 o'clock on a Saturday night.

The attending listens to Michael nonjudgmentally and then says, "Try to detach yourself from the immediacy of the situation. [Note how empathy involves distance as well as closeness.] Pretend you are invisible and looking down at the interaction between the two of you from a spot on the ceiling. Forget about yourself; watch that guy named Michael down there. Ask yourself: Why is it that Johnnie might be reacting with such hostility to Michael? Give her the benefit of the doubt. At least *try* to see it from her point of view. What do you come up with?"

"Well," Michael muses, "she seems determined to prove that she's the one in control. She is filled with so much anger."

"True. What else?" the attending prods.

"Well," Michael continues, "there's no doubt that she's putting me down. She's trying to make me feel like two cents."

"And succeeding. But why would she need to do a thing like that?" the attending persists.

"I remember something now," Michael says suddenly. "Just before I was going to examine her, before the intern and resident left, one of them made a pretty crude joke. Something about her partner keeping "watch" while she "worked." She laughed it off, but I could tell she was hurt. I think she even blushed a little, but they were already leaving the room.

"Then you came in," the attending notes.

"Right. Maybe they hurt her pride?"

"Maybe she was making *you* feel as humiliated and inadequate as they had just made *her* feel!"

"I can understand now why she reacted that way toward me."

"So what do you say now?" the attending asks.

"I don't know. What would you say?"

The attending obliges. "Agree with her."

Michael looked bewildered.

"Agree with her." the attending repeats. "Empathize with her plight. Not only is she insulted and degraded, but on top of that they send a junior medical student in to do her history and physical."

"Well," Michael says somewhat skeptically, "I'll give it a try."

Roll the camera to action—scene 1, take 2.

Michael approaches the bed again. Johnnie still sits there, a contemptuous scowl on her face. This time, however, Michael notices something else—something sadder, a weariness and vulnerability this tough woman tries hard to hide.

"I'm Michael Smith, a junior medical student. Has Dr. Jones explained that I need to get a history and physical from you?"

"How old are you anyway?!" Johnnie starts in, "No way is a student experimenting on me!"

Michael bites his lips this time and gives the new approach a try.

"You're not having much luck around here, are you?" he begins. "It's bad enough to be sick and have to go to the county ward, but on *top* of that, they send in a scut monkey to examine you—a junior medical student. I'd be upset, too!"

Johnnie looks momentarily nonplussed, then her expression softens. "Well, I guess you kids have it hard, too. You've got to start somewhere."

"I think it's important for you to know," Michael says, "I'll be the one taking care of you. The other doctors are also going to be monitoring you. I'm very concerned about this pain you've been having."

"Ah, what the hell," Johnnie says. "What do you wanna know?"

Clearly, we could have bypassed this lengthy dissection of the empathic process by simply saying, "Put yourself in the patient's shoes," or "Empathize but don't identify." Yet, such admonitions, nice as they sound, seldom help a great deal. To make sense of it, one needs to look at the process in more detail. Several themes emerge when we do:

1. A breakdown in empathy usually begins when a patient pulls the doctor's chain. The specifics can vary, but patients are good at it. In Michael's case, the patient misdirected her anger and lashed out at Michael, who was vulnerable to attacks on his youth and inexperience. Other patients can, and do, throw other kinds of brickbats—seductiveness, hostility, passivity, demandingness, and more.
2. The empathic bond ruptures further when the doctor assumes the attack on him is based on objective reality. This prevents him from asking, "Why does the patient feel compelled to see me like this?" Instead, the doctor becomes defensive and feels compelled to disprove the validity of the patient's attack. This approach rarely succeeds. Typically, a doctor first redoubles his efforts to be kind, smart, wise—whatever the patient is accusing him of being deficient in. When this fails, as it almost always does, the doctor then typically responds with increased authoritarianism and hostility.
3. This completes a self-fulfilling prophecy in which the doctor becomes the very person the patient fears.
4. As this case shows, empathy requires the doctor almost literally be in several places at once. If the doctor is insensitive to the painful messages the patient is sending out in the first place, he will never be able to understand the patient's real anguish.

He *must* feel the pain the patient intends him to feel. At the same time, he must be able to detach himself from the immediate situation and realize that what is being directed toward him comes more from the fact that he is a symbol than from any reality that has to do with him.
5. Although achieving this kind of equanimity can be difficult, it permits the physician to speak sincerely "over his patient's shoulder," so to speak, so that the cliché, "Being in the patient's shoes," takes on real meaning.

Empathy is one of the hardest skills to perfect. It is also one of our most effective tools. Nothing is foolproof, of course, but most situations that go awry do so from lack of empathy. Even enormously explosive situations can often be defused with accurate empathy. Obviously, the uses of empathy are not limited to understanding patients. One can also use empathy better to understand the complex and sometimes painful interactions that occur among various hospital personnel, including ourselves.

One final point: Note that oversimplified prescriptions for actions and interventions are downplayed throughout this text. Students do, understandably, find the absence of such prescriptions frustrating. However, despite students' understandable wishes for specific courses of action, remedies, or antidotes, we have chosen to refrain. It is our contention that the student who truly accepts the patient and empathizes with the patient's plight *will* know what action to take and when to take it. Other books may offer easy "tricks of the trade" and recipes for sure-fire success. Although these cookbooks reduce anxiety momentarily, they ultimately ring hollow. Patient-centered medicine is simply too complex. The proper intervention must come from true understanding and empathy. When these are achieved, what to do usually arises naturally. Without understanding and empathy, no lexicon of tricks or list of techniques will succeed.

## Conceptualization

The conceptual basis for patient-centered medicine that we advocate is derived from George Engel's biopsychosocial model described in Chapters 2 and 3. Essentially, Engel's thesis is based on principles of systems theory and holds that no change can occur within one component of a system without eventually making an impact on other components of that system. Further, each system (eg, a molecule, a human being, a family) holds a lower or higher place in relation to other systems in a hierarchy of systems. Approaching patient care from this perspective requires a shift in thinking away from a simplistic disease orientation toward the more complex and more effective stance that we describe here as patient-centered medicine. The following two chapters, which describe the theoretical basis of this approach in greater detail, underscore how difficult a challenge it is to make this shift in perspective. To be a good doctor, a truly complete one, physicians must understand molecules and cells, organelles and organs, but they must also understand the complex, ineffable miracle we call "the person." Even this will not suffice, however; for as Engel's diagrams make clear, people relate primarily in dyads but live in still larger systems—families, communities, and the biosphere itself.

Once upon a time, being a doctor must have seemed easier. Now it is more challenging than before. The onslaught of new information at all levels of the systems hierarchy has accelerated at an astonishing rate. These are not trivial advances, but major new trends, fundamental and far-reaching discoveries doctors must integrate and understand.

A man who loses his business has a heart attack. Six months later, he dies. Long ago we would have attributed it to coincidence. Now an increasing body of evidence tells us otherwise. Farmers in Montana spray insecticide over a wheat field. A month later, poisoned waterfowl in 30 states endanger the entire food chain. Advances in biomolecular technology will give you pause—from a group of scientists who cloned the first mammal successfully, Dolly the sheep, from an adult somatic cell to groundbreaking research in gene-editing technology to the early stages of pharmacogenomics and its role in personalized medicine. Their far-reaching effects resonate through the entire system of humankind all the way to the most fundamental ethical and spiritual tenets of civilization.

What are conscientious doctors to do? Students are already overwhelmed with the amount of new knowledge to be mastered. The mind reels with emotional and intellectual vertigo at the prospect of encompassing so much more.

What most doctors do to solve this dilemma is to draw a box around an area of relative "expertise." They do not go into primary care, where we face such a shortage in meeting the health needs of the growing population. Instead, they put a perimeter around some section of the huge and momentous total picture. The physician workforce of today leans toward specializing, and resting comfortably within the specific scope of practice.

The biases, misconceptions, and prejudices that accompany all territoriality emerge (once you have drawn your box, you have defined what is, and is not, in your territory). Take, for example, a general practitioner (GP) who inherits a patient with migraine headaches who has been taking long-term opioids for analgesia prescribed by her former doctor. Assessments and investigations completed by the GP are inconclusive; meanwhile, the patient demands relief for her pain. A referral to neurology is made, although declined given the cause is conjectured to be from medication overuse. The advice is to taper the patient off opioids and refer her to a pain specialist. A referral to the pain service is made, although declined given the etiology of the headaches needs to be investigated fully first—by neurology. And we come to an impasse, with the patient left to suffer if the GP does not yield to what the patient has only known to relieve the pain. The GP is left in a bind given her knowledge about the harms of long-term opioid use, but without input from specialists, she cannot offer an alternative.

Moving into the realm of the teaching environment, on a practical day-to-day basis, typical junior and senior medical students learn their box is being drawn at the organ system level. It is difficult enough to endure the rigors of a typical admitting night. The nuances of acid–base balance, pharmacotherapy, and electrocardiophysiology seem staggering. Who has time for even these critical matters, let alone subjects more encompassing of the entire human condition?

Reluctantly, somewhat uneasily, somewhere during the clinical years typical students are tempted to turn their back on the larger problems of their patients. They say, implicitly if not explicitly, "I do not hear. It's not that I don't want to hear. It's just that I can't afford to hear. Not right now, anyway, not for the next few years."

Obviously, we have no simple solutions, but we can offer a general principle: Do not expect the impossible of yourself. If students and doctors can learn to accept ambiguity, learn to live with the lack of mastery that is inevitable during any period of knowledge explosion; self-reflect on your limitations and when to seek input. It may still be possible to embrace a broader view of patient care—one that modern medicine clearly demands.

It is *not* necessary to be an expert at every level of the total ecosystem to be a good doctor. It is presumptuous to try and impossible to succeed. What we do need to begin to appreciate more is the way things fit together as well as the infinite manners in which they fall apart. We have gotten a better education in dissecting sick people than we have in appreciating how healthy people stay harmonious and whole.

In "The Silken Tent," Robert Frost wrote:

> She is as in a field a silken tent
> At midday when a sunny summer breeze
> Has dried the dew and all its ropes relent,
> So that in guys it gently sways at ease,
> And its supporting central cedar pole,
> That is its pinnacle to be heavenward
> And signifies the sureness of the soul,
> Seems to owe naught to any single cord,
> But strictly held by none, is loosely bound
> By countless silken ties of love and thought
> To everything on earth the compass round,
> And only by one's going slightly taut
> In the capriciousness of summer air
> Is of the slightest bondage made aware.

Frost was talking about the interdependency of all humankind, yet the metaphor also extends to medicine. Instead of quarreling, if not coexisting at arm's length from the safety of our theoretical boxes, we must begin to appreciate that medicine as a human experience involves all of us at all levels of the systems hierarchy, embracing "everything on earth the compass round." Each of us, with our own legitimate expertise, must begin to realize we are all strands linked by a silken tent woven from the fabric of our shared humanness.

This is a very simple notion, yet one that is heeded too rarely. To medical students, we say: As you dig your way through the mountains of facts, beware of those who burrow their own little holes in those mountains and then growl at approaching strangers. We are all miners.

Patient-centered medicine is not easy. The real challenge of the biopsychosocial model comes from its demand that doctors view patients both so broadly and in such depth. It demands, above all, perspective, whereby doctors try to understand both themselves and their patients, and how things fit together, instead of all the artificial and pathological ways they can be induced to fall apart—from self-destructiveness and despair to the ravages of the disease process itself. Good patient care requires an integrative perspective.

The following vignette of two physicians' trekking excursion in Nepal offers such insight. Uyen and her friend Kim Le, an integrative psychiatrist in Santa Barbara, endured a harrowing night afflicted by altitude sickness on the Annapurna trail, an illness trekkers may plan for adequately but can nonetheless strike unpredictably. Uyen's story is juxtaposed upon Kim's, both witnessing each other's fears and coming away with different experiences. Here is Uyen's recollection of that night:

> Thinking back to that sleepless night in Ghorepani, where we would lay camp in a modest teahouse after a long, strenuous day of hiking, the felt sense was of helplessness, feeling ill-prepared for the insidious effects of altitude sickness. It was a cold, wet evening in April 2014, at the end of day 2 of our trek, with the highlight to summit at Poon Hill within reach. I had experienced fatigue, breathlessness, and nausea, which I assumed were within the normal range of physical symptoms expected from the rigors of a varying gradual and steep trek the Nepalese described as "a little bit up and a little bit down." Although Kim and I were reasonably fit, with some preacclimatization training above the expected highest peak on our trek, we had underestimated the toll such a rapid ascent exacted on us physically and mentally. We ascended nearly 5500 feet in 2 days, from Nayapul to Ghorepani. As part of a commercial group, we adhered to a tight time schedule that did not phase the rest of our group. Nor did it phase us until 48 hours into the trek, typically when symptoms of altitude sickness emerge.
>
> The highlight of the trek was nearly upon us—to reach Poon Hill early the next morning in hopes of catching the sunrise amid the snowcapped, rugged peaks of the Himalayas. Poon Hill stood at approximately 10 500 feet in contrast to Ghorepani, at around 9 100 feet, both "slight" in comparison with elevations along the circuit rising up to 15 000 feet. Our trek was in the minor league. We were not alongside ambitious mountaineers with sights on Everest or K2. Our group ranged from avid hikers from Europe and America to a retired Swiss couple in their 60s—novice hikers, one of whom (the wife of the Swiss couple) smoked regularly throughout the trek. This retired pair kept up with the leisurely half of our group, which included Kim and I, and even finished ahead of us.
>
> Our trek would have been impossible without porters, hard-working Nepalese men who did the work of giants. They were tasked with carrying gear as heavy as 30 kg, and they still finished ahead of us, then doubling back graciously to check in and guide the remaining way. Quiet and unassuming, they followed alongside us—alongside these women who appeared fit, yet struggled to maintain the group's pace. We were the last to finish both days, in part a result of admiring the beauty of our surroundings and in part a delay by increasing fatigue and breathlessness.
>
> It did not occur to me we were experiencing altitude sickness until we checked our oxygen saturation using a pulse oximeter. My oxygen sats were repeatedly in the low 90s. Kim's fell below this, and was complicated by tachypnea and tachycardia. My suffering paled in comparison with hers. The carefree spirit of my friend

was diminished, overshadowed by a languid body whose vitals struggled to compensate. I was deeply troubled, having never seen my friend that unwell.

The most effective treatment for altitude sickness is to descend, but it was late evening. The only route down in the dark, unlit night was by way of medical evacuation. There was not even supplemental oxygen on site, as medical resources were scarce. We had acetazolamide, knew of its indication (and mixed outcome anecdotally), and decided against it. Some may call it foolish, but the thought of polyuria with repeated trips to the outdoor toilet in the middle of a miserably chilly night when our bodies were leaden from fatigue was beyond tolerable.

Gopal, the lead guide for our trek, was seasoned, having led his men to much higher summits through countless treks many years over—someone who earned quickly the trust and respect from our group. His advice, delivered in a measured way that belied a tone of uncertainty, was simply to keep watch and wait until the next day to descend by pony. I thought otherwise and urged Kim to err on the side of caution, to call for a medical evacuation. She did not weigh her decision lightly. Kim considered her expectations for the trip on balance with what she knew about the environment, about her health status, and about her own capabilities to heal. She firmly declined medical evacuation and, nervously, I respected her decision.

So I lay in a tattered bunk across from her, just keeping watch, the shallow rise and fall of her chest and soft sounds of her breathing. In her quiet way, she tried to reassure me of her ability to stabilize her vitals through inducing a trance state. Hearing this from anyone else would have raised skepticism, but Kim has trained in a diverse range of evidence-based practices. I trusted her, but did not have trust in the unknowns of our environment. I felt helpless, offering what seemed like meager support and empty words. As I struggled to stay awake, fatigue eventually eclipsed my fears, and sleep settled upon me. It was the longest night of my adult life.

Early the next morning, I opened my eyes to see Kim sleeping peacefully and breathing comfortably. I tapped her gently and she awoke slowly. It was a surreal moment, as if in one fell swoop, her awaking erased the dreadful events of the night before. I didn't have much to say, just feeling tremendous relief and being so thankful my friend made it through the long, cold night. She had no intention of summiting that morning, and in her selfless way, encouraged me to go. I left her, reluctantly, to rest—my caring friend who, even when seized by illness, possessed the capacity to be considerate of others.

After Poon Hill, we found each other at breakfast and sat quietly, taking in our surroundings one last time. Kim's strength was slow to return, but her spirit rebounded quickly. As our group descended, she followed behind us trotting away by pony, and smiling as she took in the majesty of the Himalayas.

To this day, the uncertainty of her survival and feelings of helplessness remain with me in a palpable way whenever I reflect back to that sleepless night. I remain awestruck by Kim's composure, as she was acting as both patient and physician, using hypnotherapy to stabilize her vitals, and providing me solace before resigning to acceptance. She epitomizes the humanistic physician.

The following story in Kim's words:

We made it. After 10 hours of trekking we arrived at the gates of Ghorepani. Perfect timing as well. The winds were picking up; the sky darkened ominously as the gray clouds gathered. Then, the first raindrops started falling. We had just enough time to pull up the hood of our jacket to cover our head and take a couple of quick photos at the gate to document our triumphant arrival. The drizzle became a steady rain very quickly. As exhausted as I was, there was a second wind of energy that propelled me forward to the teahouse, fueled by the elation of being so close to finishing today's trek and the desire to be sheltered indoors away from the chilly, gusty wind and rain. At some point I no longer felt my body consciously. There was just seeing, hearing, smelling, and thoughts. It took at least another 20 minutes to ascend to our teahouse, where we met up with the rest of our trekking group. I saw familiar faces and managed to smile, but engaging in conversation seemed to require too much effort. I remained mostly silent—an observing, disembodied shadow following Uyen around. We went to our room to rest. I allowed myself to start registering various bodily sensations again, such as the pins-and-needles sensations in my extremities, the headache and nausea; my whole body felt like a quivering mass of Jell-O, unable to support its own weight as I plopped myself down on the bed. My nose felt congested and started running. I found a Kleenex and wiped it, noticing bright red blood. We rested for some time on our beds and, looking over at Uyen, I could tell she was also exhausted. It was time for dinner but I had no appetite nor the energy to drag myself out of bed. I could see the look of concern on Uyen's face. Not knowing what to do, she asked me if there was anything she could do to help me feel better—such a simple gesture that conveys powerfully both empathy and validation of my discomfort. I think many of us, including myself, tend to forget how incredibly healing and comforting that simple gesture is until we find ourselves in that situation. I replied that some ginger tea would be helpful and she proceeded to ensure attentively that my water bottle always had some ginger tea in it for the rest of the night without me having to ask a second time. I cannot emphasize enough how powerfully therapeutic these simple acts of kindness are to the human psyche. Similar to the child who gets her scraped knee kissed by her mother, the sting and burn may linger, but the suffering has dissipated entirely through a loving gesture of acknowledgment. The compassion and attentiveness that Uyen provided was, in itself, a healing salve. Although we faced uncertainty, it was reassuring to know she was always there for me. That was more than enough.

Later in the evening, Gopal, our guide, stopped by our room to check on me. He had his pulse oximeter with him. He took a few readings that indicated my resting pulse was in the high 150s/low 160s and my oxygen saturation ranged in the high 80s to low 90s. I could see the look of concern on Uyen's face intensifying and bordering on panic. I was dismayed by the readings and thought I had done a better job of training for this trek, having gone on frequent, long hikes with steep inclines. I wondered whether having the pulmonary and liver arteriovenous malformations from hereditary hemorrhagic telengiectasia put me at increased risk for altitude sickness. Was that the reason for the absurd readings? The three of us discussed my options: med-evac or be carried by pony to the next stop at lower elevation. Uyen thought it would be more prudent for me to be med-evacuated. I cannot say I am the most prudent person. Furthermore, I knew that as long as I was able to get to a lower elevation and have some time to rest, then I would be fine. I did not want to have to miss out on the rest of the trek. We made arrangements for me to be carried by pony the next morning. After Gopal left, I checked my pulse again using the stopwatch on my phone. Still in the high 150s. I knew I had to lower my heart rate; otherwise, I could go into high output heart failure. Uyen expressed her concerns and brought up the possibility of a med-evac again. I could see how worried she was, the look of helplessness on her face. My heart went out to her. She appeared to be in much more distress than I was. I would have switched places with her if I could. Although I had some physical discomfort and overwhelming fatigue, I also knew that the suffering caused by anxiety and feelings of helplessness can be much worse than any physical pain. I do not know why I was not more worried or afraid at that time. Perhaps I was too fatigued and did not have the energy. Perhaps it was also because I knew that I had someone I can trust, like Uyen, by my side.

There was nothing left to do but to surrender myself to the moment, which I found to be quite peaceful. It was like coming home—a familiar state I have discovered through meditation over the years. It occurred to me that I could hypnotize myself to lower my heart rate. I reassured Uyen regarding my hypnotic abilities and told her that I would be fine. I was confident of it. I proceeded to hypnotize myself and my heart rate dropped gradually to 110 beats per minute at resting. I reassured her that my heart rate was already improving. She appeared somewhat relieved, but I could still see the worry lingering. I tried to reassure her the best I could. She needed to get her rest for the long trek tomorrow, rather than waste her energy worrying about me. I went into a deeper state of absorption and stillness to lower my heart rate further and conserve my energy. Uyen continued to check on me throughout the night, and although I could hear her moving during the night, I was in such a deep state of absorption I could not move or speak to indicate to her that I was alright. Morning came and I broke from my trance state. I imagine it to be similar to what bears might feel when coming out of hibernation—weak and hungry, but at least my appetite was back. During breakfast, we both admired how the Annapurna mountain range looked, set against the backdrop of the early morning sun.

Although Kim and I have talked about this night in depth, I have trouble, to this day, accepting that I provided her great comfort, given my own perceived failings of not being able to do more. Although short of medical evacuation, which she did not want, "more" was simply staying attuned, respecting her wishes, and providing comfort measures. Kim's courage and composure in the face of a potentially destabilizing situation are reflective of the human spirit.

The observant student will note that Engel's diagrams in Chapter 2 consider "the biosphere" as the most encompassing unit in the systems hierarchy. We believe there is still another dimension. Whether one calls it spirit, religion, the existential nature of life—questions about the meaning of life—some order seems to prevail in the universe. In saying this, we do not wish to foist our view on anyone. However, we feel the need to expand the biopsychosocial model to a more broadly encompassing biopsychosocialspiritual approach—or, as articulated by Dr. Weil in his Foreword, to an integrative approach to consider all these dimensions.

We are troubled by contemporary medicine's lack of appreciation for the human spirit. Where is our awe when we contemplate the mystery and miracle of life itself? For ourselves, this sense of awe has brought us our greatest moments of transcendence, peace, and lucidity in settings that would otherwise depress, frighten, and elicit unremitting despair. Somehow, there have been precious moments that justify all our strivings, when the endless knowledge that we have had to absorb, the unrelenting ambiguity of our work, the impossibility of ever knowing all that we want and need to know have truly been worth it. At special moments, a remarkable clarity has emerged, and at these moments we have felt fulfilled and serene.

We appreciate that many will not relate to our own views, and this is fine. Yet even if students do not see the relevance of such a perspective for themselves, they need to realize how important spiritual concerns are for many of their patients. There is emerging evidence on the role of spirituality in health and healing.[22] The prevailing ethos of contemporary medicine may not necessarily refuse the importance of spiritual concerns, but it is neglected in formal education[23] and broadly not queried routinely by even the most discerning clinicians.

## Competence

In concluding the four basic principles of patient-centered medicine, it seems appropriate to end with competence. Ultimately, knowledge and intellect alone are not sufficient to make one a good doctor, but neither are compassion and empathy alone. We are dealing with live patients, real people who place themselves in our hands. What we do or do not do can make the difference between life and death, recovery and degeneration, health and illness. Even if we do not cause disability or death to a patient through gross incompetence (what students dread), ultimately it is our competence that determines the quality of our patients' lives on countless levels.

Allow us to return once more to Johnnie, our suffering patient with alcoholism. If Michael had not been able to empathize with her, Johnnie would not have died as a result. However, the insensitivity would have left another small wound, one more tiny cut in a lifetime of slashes and piercing misfortunes. Today's physician demands competence in this regard, and Michael would have been incompetent to ignore the sensitive nature of her social situation. At the same time, Michael's empathy alone would not have been enough to ensure competence. He also must understand how to work up an acute abdomen. He must know how to formulate a good differential diagnosis. Johnnie could have had alcoholic pancreatitis, as everyone suspected, but also she could have had a stone in her common duct, pancreatic carcinoma, even myocardial disease. The list is long, and Michael must learn it to be competent. He must also know how to manage and treat the disease he ultimately diagnoses. He must, finally, know how to avoid the countless iatrogenic complications that treatment itself causes.

Beyond this, let us assume it was pancreatitis, and Michael's choice of treatment brought the amylase level down. Still, how competent would he and the other doctors have been if they simply sent Johnnie back onto the streets without appropriate input from social services, back into the social cauldron that fomented her self-destructiveness in the first place?

We cannot possibly be all things for all patients. We cannot even be all things for one patient. Yet competence does demand that we do many things. Above all, competence requires one to see the big picture. For Johnnie, this might include an attempt to get her into an alcohol treatment unit. Yes, we *know* it has been tried before. We must, at the very least, consider the destructive social context that contributes so heavily to her disease. Obviously, this is far from easy, but competence demands no less. Doctors who pretend stubbornly that their responsibility is limited to a narrow box drawn around Johnnie's pancreas are woefully and willfully wrong. They are incompetent. Finally, when doctors reach a patient, as Michael did Johnnie, they do something special. Perhaps it is just a touch or a look of understanding. One less tiny cut in the patient's life. A small wound that heals instead of festering. That is competence.

In closing, the following vignette by Uyen illustrates the healing nature and value of competence (as well as acceptance, empathy, and conceptualization) in the human experience of medical care:

> The real meaning of competence was brought home to me on a very personal level during summer 2014. I had decided that year to be free of corrective lenses and envisioned daily life unfettered from contacts or glasses. I researched different types of corrective eye surgeries and decided laser-assisted in situ keratomileusis (LASIK) most suited me, based primarily on the shorter recovery time. And, I have known many who underwent LASIK without complications.
>
> LASIK is such a common procedure that some of my friends were surprised by the amount of time I spent researching eye surgeons. There were established LASIK clinics in the Los Angeles and Orange County areas that were only in the business of laser refractive procedures, and thus offered very competitive rates. As tempting as this was, I opted for a very seasoned eye surgeon who hailed from a family of ophthalmologists, whose practice provided total eye care, and who was connected to academic medicine and involved in teaching resident eye physicians the latest surgical techniques.
>
> At my LASIK consultation, I was impressed by Dr. Leif Hertzog's gentle, empathic manner and ability to gain rapport in a relatively short interview. Assumptions were not made on why I desired LASIK, although perhaps they were obvious to others. Dr. Hertzog made a genuine inquiry to understand my reasons for this elective surgery. My examination revealed dry eyes, which in some cases may rule out LASIK. I was advised to wait a short period to see if this could be remedied with an increased use of lubricant eye drops and punctal plugs. I was a little impatient because I had an international trip planned and had wanted to undergo the procedure well before the trip.
>
> In the hectic frenzy of balancing work and my personal life, as well as planning for my trip abroad, I tried to make a case for the LASIK procedure to be moved up right before my trip, despite knowing the less than optimal healing conditions. An exception was not made because it would have rendered me vulnerable during

the recovery period. Patient-centered medicine did not mean yielding to what I cared about carte blanche, as was demonstrated here. Rather, the decision was collaborative—listening respectfully to what I valued with accurate empathy, although adhering firmly to what would provide an optimal course of recovery. I was disappointed, but respected the decision.

I entrusted Dr. Hertzog with the delicate task of enhancing my vision. He has an ability to articulate a complex procedure with simplicity and clarity. As Bill Gates once said, "If you can't explain something simply, you don't really understand it." Dr. Hertzog clearly understood and possessed both knowledge and technical expertise.

On the day of surgery, I was anxious and apprehensive, despite it being a fairly low-risk and common procedure. Complications are considered rare, I reminded myself. The procedure itself was uneventful. Anesthetic drops were applied to numb the site. Dr. Hertzog talked me through the process of creating a corneal flap, the laser remodeling of the corneal stroma, and the repositioning of the flap. After the procedure, I was armed with a kit of dark shades, antibiotic and anti-inflammatory eye drops, and instructions on when to seek urgent medical attention.

A good friend drove me home, picked up some Texas style BBQ (a treat in southern California), then had to return to her children. She had offered for me to stay with her family, but I preferred my own space and did not wish to impose. In the hours that ensued, I had a visceral experience that something was terribly wrong. I felt helpless, afraid, although reluctant to call on friends. Some discomfort was expected, but I was experiencing excruciating periorbital pain. My vision remained blurry and sensitive to light as expected, but I underestimated how disabled I would be managing on my own. I stumbled around in the kitchen, frustrated when I struggled to open the container of brisket, never mind using a fork to feed myself. This simple task I took for granted was exasperating, so I just gave up on food that night.

The pain subsided marginally, but I resisted calling my doctor or practice nurse. Reflecting back, I wonder about the hesitation that deterred me from reaching out—as if such an act meant full surrendering and dependency. Ironically, as part of acceptance (of being unwell), I would expect and encourage my patients to reach out for help when needed. It required less effort to take analgesics and go to bed early, so I reassured myself that complications are rare, rationalizing the experience as perhaps having a low threshold for pain and discomfort.

I awoke the next day nearly pain free. Opening my eyes I was pleasantly surprised to see with greater overall clarity, although some blurriness remained. I arrived at my ophthalmologist's office for the postop day 1 check, expecting a blessing for a good bill of health and medical clearance to return to work. What followed was a month-long ordeal of the uncertainty we speak about in medicine, but uncertainty experienced as a patient.

During my eye examination, central corneal opacities were present and other features were not consistent with a healthy postoperative clinical picture. My inner voice said, "There have been more than 10 million LASIK surgeries done in the

United States and complications are rare." This fact no longer provided me comfort, as panic set in regarding the reality of the situation. I had experienced a complication. In the many, many years of doing LASIK and eye surgeries, Dr. Hertzog had never encountered such a case as mine. I was speechless and just listened to him. He assured me the preoperative and operative processes did not break from standard procedure. He spoke of serious conditions to rule out. I could tell this experience, our shared experience, was quite humbling for him. An acceptance of the unknown coupled with composure in communicating the next steps based on his conceptualization eased my own anxiety.

Dr. Hertzog provided a differential of diagnoses, ruling out potential eye emergencies (ie, loss of vision). Diffuse lamellar keratitis and an infectious process were high on the differential, given a delay of treatment could be disastrous, so I remained on prophylactic steroid and antibiotic ophthalmic drops. Dr. Hertzog referred me to a cornea specialist, a colleague he trusted and who was on faculty at the academic institution with which he was affiliated. Competence was evidenced by a self-awareness of his limitations and urgency in seeking specialist input.

Within 1 week, I was evaluated by 2 cornea specialists affiliated with 2 major academic medical institutions in Los Angeles. The first specialist was confident in making the diagnosis. She suspected I had central toxic keratopathy (CTK), a rare syndrome on which she had written a textbook chapter. It was so rare she had never seen a case until I had presented. One large, prospective study cited the incidence of CTK was 0.016% of 6131 eyes that undergone LASIK.[24] The same day she examined me, she consulted another cornea specialist who had originally described CTK as a distinct syndrome from diffuse lamellar keratitis. She spotted something concerning in the stroma of my right eye—a small chance it could be an evolving necrotic process. She maintained a high index of suspicion and referred me. Off I went to see the second cornea specialist in his Beverly Hills office. I was beside myself but managed to suppress my emotions; emotions that later found their way to the surface when I was still enough to reflect.

Brevity was to be expected when the second cornea specialist arrived at his busy practice. He had just come from surgery and my visit was unscheduled, kindly agreed upon as a collegial request. He was polite, professional, and simply got to the point. At that moment, what I valued most was his technical expertise. He was confident my situation was not an evolving necrotic process. He confirmed it was CTK, an acute and self-limited syndrome with unknown etiology. I was told I could stop taking the steroid drops because I had a noninflammatory process, and that my vision would not get worse, nor better, on its own. He noted that any residual hyperopia could be treated successfully in the future with an enhancement laser procedure.

He was the expert in the field in this regard, and had retreated a handful of patients with CTK successfully. I assured him I had zero desire to return for any laser procedure unless it was life-saving. And, as if reading what lay in the recesses of my mind, he volunteered—without me asking—that Dr. Hertzog did nothing wrong, a view shared by the first cornea specialist as well. This reinforced what I had already known.

Dr. Hertzog exhibited competence on many levels, from unwavering empathy to a calm acceptance (which resonated and perhaps allowed me to reciprocate the same) to conceptualizing a plan with swiftness in the face of ambiguity. Even after CTK was confirmed and the course of recovery made known, he maintained close follow-up in addition to calling me periodically after hours to check on my progress. I was even given his personal mobile number for contact should any questions or concerns arise. I never called, but the empathic gesture was deeply appreciated and it came from a genuine place of compassion.

What is not lost on me was the fear of going blind during the many moments of holding space with the unknown. To experience uncertainty as a patient in a sudden, unexpected turn, provided valuable perspective I cannot take for granted. Technical competence alone would not have been enough, nor would compassion in the absence of technical expertise. Both were essential—a vital balance. Dr. Hertzog was not an expert on all levels of the biopsychosocial system, as he need not be. It was clear he grasped the system while accepting and relating to his patient, which is no small achievement. Somehow, he understood "the silken tent."

## SUMMARY

In this initial chapter, we outlined four guiding principles of medicine as a human experience: acceptance, empathy, conceptualization, and competence. Acceptance and empathy are essential to developing a healing partnership with one's patients. Both stem from self-awareness, for it is difficult to accept another human being if you have not first accepted yourself. Conceptualization, using the biopsychosocial model and even expanding it to include issues of existential meaning and the human spirit, is related directly to comprehensive medical care; it also relates integrally to our fourth principle: competence. It is our belief that if students develop and adhere to these precepts during medical school, they will not only become better physicians, but also they will be more inwardly fulfilled in their choice of a career. These principles emphasize we are all part of the human family. Osler implied as much more than nearly a century ago when he stated that a medical degree entitled physicians to a life-long education in two spheres: the inner and the special. He spoke of the necessity of aspiring to both: (1) inner education, a knowledge of one's self; and (2) special education, a knowledge of medicine. Osler also understood the importance of the human spirit, for he admonished physicians always to "mix the waters of science with the oil of faith." Shifting metaphors somewhat, we add: Into the bedrock of your hard-won technical knowledge let the tendrils of hope and compassion at long last take root; let the seeds of your humanity and love finally germinate and grow.

## REFERENCES

1. Reiser DE, Rosen DH. *Medicine as a Human Experience*. Rockville: Aspen Publication; 1984.
2. Kohn LT, Corrigan JM, Donaldson MS, eds. *To Err Is Human: Building a Safer Health System*. Committee on Quality of Health Care in America, Institute of Medicine. Washington, DC: National Academy Press; 2000.
3. Committee on Quality of Health Care in America. *Crossing the Quality Chasm: A New Health System for the 21st Century*. Institute of Medicine. Washington, DC: National Academy Press; 2001.
4. Agency for Healthcare Research and Quality staff. *The Six Domains of HealthCare Quality*. Rockville, MD: Agency for Healthcare Research and Quality. Content last reviewed March 2016. http://www.ahrq.gov/professionals/quality-patient-safety/talkingquality/create/sixdomains.html. Accessed December 2, 2016.
5. Committee on the Health Professions Education Summit Board on Health Care Services. *Health Professions Education: A Bridge to Quality*. Institute of Medicine. Washington, DC: National Academy Press; 2003.
6. Carraccio C, Wolfsthal SD, Englander R, Ferentz K, Martin C. Shifting paradigms: from Flexner to competencies. *Acad Med*. 2002;77(5):361–367.
7. Batalden P, Leach D, Swing S, Dreyfus H, Dreyfus S. General competencies and accreditation in graduate medical education: An antidote to overspecification in the education of medical specialists. *Health Aff*. 2002;21:103–111.
8. Swing SR. The ACGME outcome project: retrospective and prospective. *Med Teach*. 2007;29:648–654.
9. Holmboe ES, Edgar L, Hamstra S. *The Milestones Guidebook*. Version 2016. http://www.acgme.org/Portals/0/MilestonesGuidebook.pdf. Accessed August 14, 2016.
10. Philibert I, Patow C, Cichon J. Incorporating patient- and family-centered care into resident education: approaches, benefits, and challenges. *J Grad Med Educ*. 2011; 272–278.
11. Committee on the Governance and Financing of Graduate Medical Education; Board on Health Care Services. *Graduate Medical Education That Meets the Nation's Health Needs*. Institute of Medicine. Washington, DC: National Academy Press; 2014.
12. Association of American Medical College staff. *Optimizing: A Five-Year Road Map for America's Medical Schools, Teaching Hospitals, and Health Systems*. Washington, DC: Association of American Medical Colleges; 2015. https://www.aamc.org/download/425468/data/optimizinggmereport.pdf. Accessed December 2, 2016.
13. Kirch DB, Mitchell K, Ast C. The new 2015 MCAT: testing competencies. *JAMA*. 2013;310(21):2243–2244.
14. Association of American Medical College staff. *Core Competencies of Entering Medical Students*. Association of American Medical College. https://www.aamc.org/initiatives/admissionsinitiative/competencies. Accessed August 14, 2016.
15. Mead N, Bowers P. Patient-centredness: a conceptual framework and review of the empirical literature. *Soc Sci Med*. 2000;51(7):1081–110.
16. Stewart M. Evidence for the patient-centered clinical method as a means of implementing the biopsychosocial approach. In: Frankel RM, Quill TE, McDaniel SH, eds. *The Biopsychosocial Approach: Past, Present, and Future*. Rochester, NY: University of Rochester Press; 2003:123–132.

17. Tronick E, Adamson LB, Als H, Brazelton TB. Infant emotions in normal and pertubated interactions. Paper presented at the biennial meeting of the Society for Research in Child Development, Denver, CO, April 1975.
18. Goldman, JG. *Thoughtful Animal: Ed Tronick and the "Still Face Experiment."* October 2010. http://scienceblogs.com/thoughtfulanimal/2010/10/18/ed-tronick-and-the-still-face. Accessed August 14, 2016.
19. Cassem NH, Hackett TP. Psychiatric consultation in a coronary care unit. *Ann Intern Med.* 1971;75:9–14.
20. Cassem NH, Hackett TP. The setting of intensive care. In: Cassem NH, Hackett TP, eds. *Massachusetts General Hospital Handbook of General Hospital Psychiatry.* St. Louis: Mosby; 1978.
21. Hojat ML, Vergare MJ, Maxwell K, et al. The devil is in the third year: a longitudinal study of erosion of empathy in medical school. *Acad Med.* 2009;84(9):1182–1191.
22. Singh DM, Ajinkya S. Spirituality and religion in modern medicine. *Indian J Psychol Med.* 2012;34:399–402.
23. Rasinski KA, Kalad YG, Yoon JD, Curlin FA. An assessment of US physicians' training in religion, spirituality, and medicine. *Med Teach.* 2011;33:944–945.
24. Jutley G, Aiello F, Robaei D, Maurino V. Central toxic keratopathy after laser in situ keratomileusis. *J Cataract Refract Surg.* 2014;40:1985–1993.

## SUGGESTED READINGS

Cassell EJ. The nature of suffering and the goals of medicine. *N Engl J Med.* 1982;306: 639–645.

Cope O. *Man, Mind and Medicine.* Philadelphia: Lippincott; 1968.

Cousins N. 1979. *Anatomy of an Illness as Perceived by the Patient: Reflection on Healing and Regeneration.* New York: Norton; 1979.

Frankyl VE. *The Doctor and the Soul.* New York: Vintage Books; 1973.

Lipp MR. *Respectful Treatment: The Human Side of Medical Care.* Hagerstown, MD: Harper & Row; 1977.

Osler W. *Aequanimitas.* London: Lewis; 1906.

Reiser DE. Struggling to stay human: one student's reflections on becoming a doctor. *New Physician.* 1973;22:295–299.

Rosen DH. Physician, heal thyself. *Clin Med.* 1973;80:25–27.

# 2

# CLINICAL APPLICATION OF THE BIOPSYCHOSOCIAL MODEL

*George L. Engel*

How physicians approach patients is very much influenced by the scientific model in which their knowledge and experience are organized. Commonly, however, physicians are largely unaware of the power that this model exerts on their thinking and behavior. This is because the model is not necessarily made explicit. Rather, it becomes that part of the fabric of education that is taken for granted, the cultural background against which they learn to become physicians. Their teachers, their mentors, the texts they use, the practices they are encouraged to follow, and even the medical institution and administrative organizations in which they work reflect the prevailing conceptual model of the era.

For many years the dominant scientific model in medicine has been what is now called the biomedical model. Its origins have been traced back to the successes of Newton's mechanistic physics in the 17th century and to the decision of established Christian orthodoxy to lift the prohibition against dissection of the human body so long as physicians agreed to limit their attention to the party and leave man's soul, morals, mind, and behavior to the Church. This compact helped determine that the scientific model of Western medicine be based on reductionism and mind–body dualism. Reductionism assumes that the understanding of a complex entity can be best achieved by identifying and analyzing its component parts, from which the whole can be reconstructed. It fosters a view that nature is composed of discrete entities interacting in a linear, causal fashion and encourages the tendency to invoke simple cause-and-effect relationships. Its influence is evident in the habit of speaking of diseases not as dynamic processes but as discrete entities. Dualism predicates separation of mind from body, of the psychological from the somatic, and provides no conceptual framework, other than reductionism, whereby the two can be related.

## LIMITS OF THE BIOMEDICAL MODEL

As a scientific framework within which to elaborate the disordered bodily mechanisms involved in disease, the biomedical model has been extraordinarily fruitful. However, its underlying reductionism and dualism have served to deflect scientific attention from the more personal, human, psychological, and social aspects of health and disease. These, biomedicine considers neither accessible to rigorous scientific evaluation nor essential for the formal education of the physician. Rather, they remain part of the "art" of medicine and of the Samaritan role of the physician, skills to be emulated but not ones possible to study or teach.

The inability of the biomedical model to include the patient and his attributes as a person, as a human being, is a crippling flaw, for in the daily work of the physician the prime objective of study is a person. Much of the data the physician utilizes are gathered within the framework of an ongoing human relationship and appear in behavioral and psychological forms, i.e. how the patient behaves and what he reports about himself and his life. This fact is not acknowledged by the biomedical model which is disease- rather than patient-oriented. It encourages a view of the patient as a machine to be repaired and the physician as the repairman. Such a perspective, as frequently caricatured in cartoons, is one source of dissatisfaction of patients.

To counter such tendencies, a model is required that permits scientific attention to the psychosocial dimensions of medicine. By "psychosocial" we refer to the whole range of psychological and social issues that are germane to health and illness and that are involved in the physician's everyday understanding and care of the patient as an individual and as a social being. They include all that heretofore has been referred to crudely as the "art" of medicine, the "bedside manner," the Samaritan and healer role of the physician, and the doctor–patient relationship. They encompass the gamut of social, cultural, and psychological processes that make for the individuality of each patient and influence susceptibility to disease and requirements for individual care. For the physician, "psychosocial" refers to a body of knowledge and a set of skills that are basic for clinical competence.

An instructive way of getting a glimpse of what is encompassed by the term "psychosocial" is to consider the complaints and expectations of the public about doctors and medical care, for it is patients and families who are the most painfully aware of what their physicians lack. Patients are the ones who tell us that doctors do not communicate well, that they do not listen, that they seem ignorant of or insensitive to personal needs and individual differences, that they often neglect the person in their zeal to pursue diagnostic and treatment procedures. They stress their physician's inaccessibility—often more indicative of the psychological remoteness of the doctor than any economic barriers or problems of geographical distance.

Attention to the criteria that patients use for illness and wellness also helps to clarify what comprises the psychosocial. Patients' criteria have to do with how one feels and how one functions: with the ability to relate, to work, to play, to struggle, to have opinions, and to make choices. For the patient, "healthy" means to be able to get on with the tasks and gratifications and to meet the challenges of life without pain, discomfort, or disability. Patients look to their physicians to know and understand them as individuals, to appreciate the significance for their health and well-being, of the conditions of their lives and living. Furthermore, they expect their physicians to have the scientific knowledge and professional competence to do so. "Psychosocial" as a frame of reference includes far more than what is ordinarily designated as "psychiatric."

The biomedical model has ill-served these requirements for physicians to meet the psychosocial needs of patients. Long overdue is a scientific model capable of encompassing these missing dimensions. The development of a general systems theory at long last provides the basis for such a new model. First applied by Weiss and von Bertalanffy to cope with the same problems in biology, this systems approach is equally appropriate for medicine. The new model is called the *biopsychosocial model*. Medicine based on the new model might be called "systems medicine."

## BIOPSYCHOSOCIAL MODEL

The advantage of the systems approach is that it provides a conceptual framework within which both organized wholes and component parts can be studied. Systems theory is best approached through the commonsense observation that nature is ordered as a hierarchically arranged continuum, with its more complex, larger units superordinate to the less complex, smaller units. This may be represented schematically by a vertical stacking to emphasize the hierarchy (Figure 2.1) and by a nest of squares to emphasize the continuum (Figure 2.2). Each level in the hierarchy represents an organized dynamic whole, a system of sufficient persistence and identity to justify being named. Cell, organ, person, family—each indicates a level of complex, integrated organization about the existence of which a high degree of consensus holds. Each system implies qualities and relationships distinctive for that level of organization, and each requires criteria for study and explanation unique for that level.

Consideration of the hierarchy as a continuum reveals another obvious fact. Each system is at the same time a component of higher systems (Figure 2.2). System *cell* is a component of systems *tissue* and *organ* and *person*. Person and *two-person* are component *family* and *community*. *In the continuity of natural systems, every unit is at the same time both a whole and a part*. Person (or individual) represents at the same time the highest level of an organismic hierarchy and the lowest level of a social hierarchy. As a whole, each system has its unique characteristics and dynamics; as the part, it is a component of a higher level system. The designation "system" refers to the existence of a stable configuration in time and space, a configuration that is maintained not only by the coordination of component parts in some kind of internal dynamic network but also by the characteristics of the larger system of which it is a part and which in turn constitutes its immediate environment. "Stable configuration" also implies the existence of boundaries between organized systems across which material and information flow. Each system is interconnected with every other system by information flow through feedback arrangements. Hence disturbances at any system level may be communicated to and affect any other system level, especially those in the closest functional relationship.

Such a systems-oriented model overcomes the limitations of dualism and reductionism and replaces the simple cause-and-effect explanations of linear causality with reciprocal causal models. Health, disease, illness, and disability can be conceptualized in terms of the relative intactness and functioning of each component system on each hierarchical level. Overall health reflects a high level of intra- and intersystemic harmony. Disruption of such harmony may be initiated at any level, be it cell, organ, person, or community. Whether the resulting disturbance is contained at the level at which it was initiated, or other levels become implicated, reflects the capacity of the initially affected system to adjust to the change, i.e. to cope. Thus a modification

30 PATIENT-CENTERED MEDICINE: A HUMAN EXPERIENCE

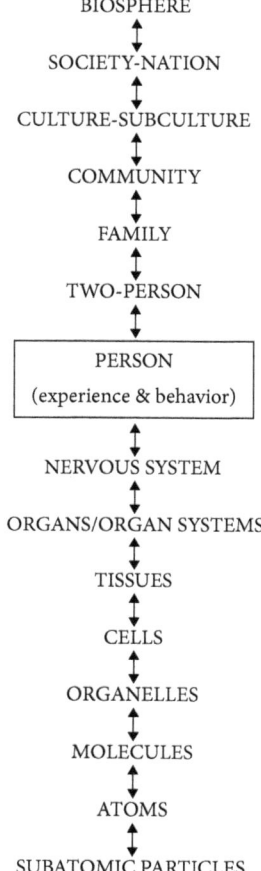

FIGURE 2.1 Systems Hierarchy: Levels of Organization

in an individual's social environment (an imposed job change, for example) impacts first on psychological functions, e.g., perceptions and appraisal. If the change is successfully accommodated at the psychological level, there will be no perceptible reverberations and other systems. For example, the individual may have no difficulty successfully handling the situation by thinking it through and resolving on a course of action—"no sweat," so to speak. Similarly, a molecular substance introduced into the body might be broken down, excreted, neutralized, or inactivated without implicating any but the particular molecular, cellular, tissue, or organ system required for its disposal. In both examples, the systems initially involved have the capacity to handle the imposed change without disruption. Under different circumstances, or in another individual with a different past history, the very same social change or the very same molecular substance may induce profound disruptions that involve many systems in

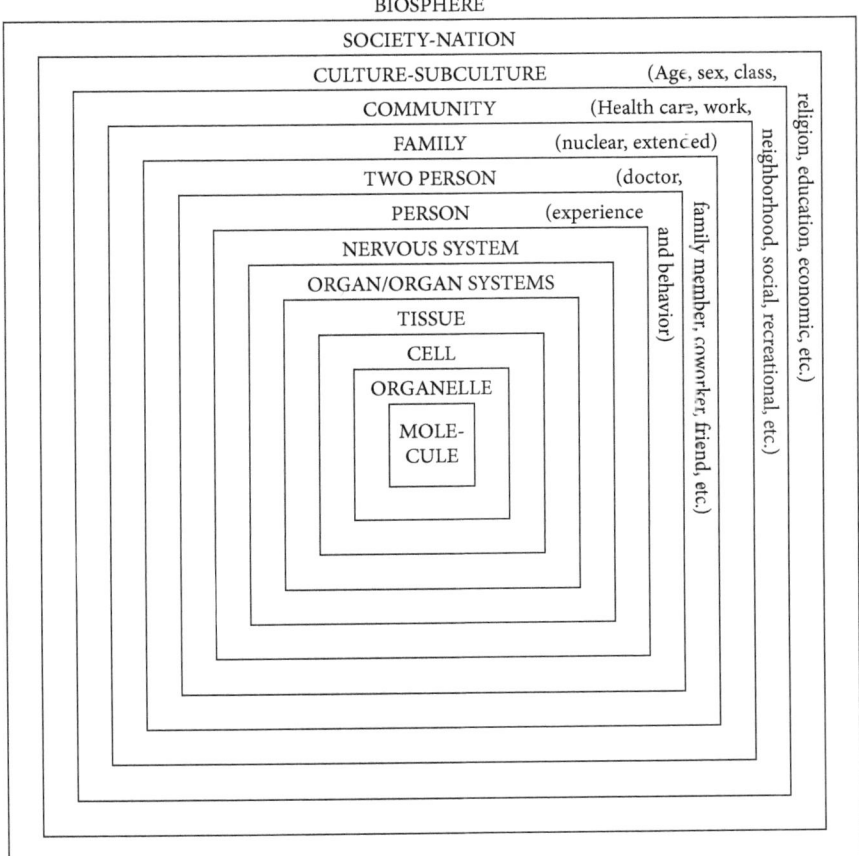

FIGURE 2.2 Biosphere

the hierarchy. Such contrasts between smooth functioning and disruption provide the basis on which health, disease, illness, and disability may be differentiated.

Central to this perspective are not only the dynamic interrelations that determine relative degrees of intra- and intersystemic harmony or disruption but also the fact that every change becomes part of the history of each system, rendering it different at each successive point in time. In the biopsychosocial model, there can be no return to the *status quo ante*. Health restored is not the same as the former state of health; it is a different intersystemic harmony than that which existed before the illness episode. Moreover, an illness not only changes the patient as an individual, it may also impact others, in the family as well as the community.

## BIOPSYCHOSOCIAL MODEL APPLIED

Let us now examine with a clinical example the application of the biopsychosocial model in everyday practice. As we said at the outset, how the physician approaches the patient is very much influenced by the scientific model he uses to organize knowledge and experience. The biopsychosocial model orients the approach in terms of the hierarchy and continuum of the natural systems that the physician must keep in mind as he undertakes the study and care of a patient.

To exemplify the systems approach, let us consider the case of Mr. Glover (a pseudonym), a 55-year-old married real estate salesman with two adult sons who was brought to the emergency department on March 1 with symptoms similar to those he had experienced 6 months earlier when he had had a myocardial infarction.

We begin consideration of the model by reminding ourselves that clinical study begins at the person level—the patient—and much of it takes place within a two-person system—the doctor–patient relationship. The data consist of reported inner experience (e.g., feelings sensations, thoughts, opinions, memories) and reported, observable behavior. From the outset, even such minimal screening data as Mr. Glover's age, gender, marital and family status, occupation, and employment already indicate system characteristics useful for future judgments and decisions. Adding to this, the information that the patient had resisted acknowledging illness (noteworthy in the face of a documented heart attack 6 months earlier) and that he had to be persuaded to seek medical attention quickly directs attention to this man's psychological style and conflicts. This alerts a systems-oriented physician to the possibility, if not the probability, that the course of the illness and the care of this patient may be importantly influenced by the processes at the psychological and interpersonal levels of organization. At the same time, the similarity of Mr. Glover's current symptoms to those of his earlier myocardial infarction directs attention to systems derangements at the cardiovascular level, not to mention the symbolic level of "another heart attack."

Such an inclusive approach, which considers all the levels of organization that might possibly be important for immediate and long-term care, may be contrasted with the parsimonious approach of the biomedical model. In the latter model, the ideal is to find as quickly as possible the simplest explanation, preferably a single diagnosis, and to regard all else as complications or as "overlay," or as just plain irrelevant to the doctor's task. For the reductionist physician, a diagnosis of "acute myocardial infarction" would suffice to characterize Mr. Glover's problem and to define the doctor's job. Thereafter, Mr. Glover would likely be referred to as "an MI," and that would be that.

By contrast, let us now reconstruct *in systems terms* the sequence of events comprising the first 90 minutes of Mr. Glover's latest episode of illness. The critical events and their consequences for intra- and intersystemic harmony are schematized in a series of diagrams (Figures 2.3 through 2.8). Each diagram indicates the systems level on which the event in question impacted, along with its reverberations up and down the systems hierarchy. Appreciating the unity of the hierarchy—that each system is at the same time also a component of higher systems—highlights the significance of the disruption of any one system for the intactness of all other systems, especially those most proximate. These interrelationships are indicated in Figures 2.3 through 2.8 by using double arrows to connect the system levels.

Figure 2.3 depicts the critical event of progressive impairment of coronary artery blood flow interrupting the oxygen supply and disrupting the organization of a segment of myocardium. Note that although changes are taking place at the levels of molecule,

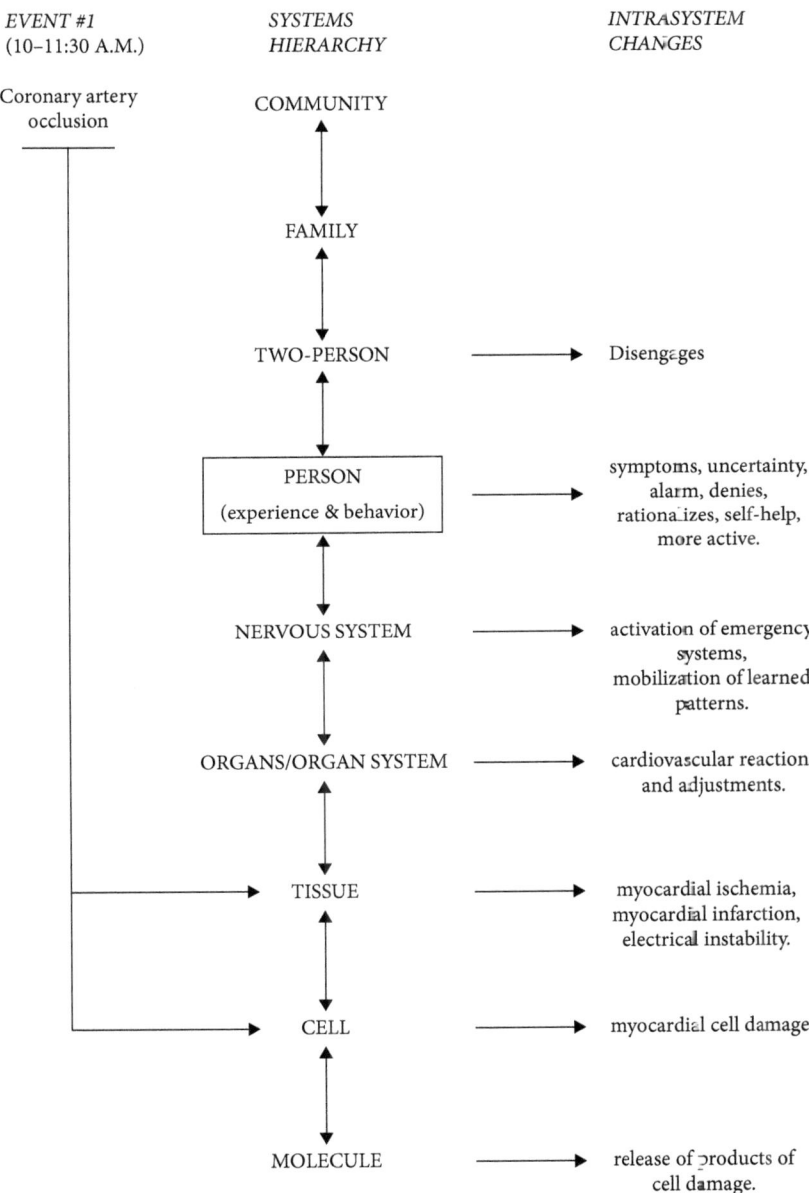

FIGURE 2.3 Biopsychosocial Model Applied

cell, tissue, organ, organ system, and nervous system, illness and patienthood do not become issues until the *person* level is implicated i.e., not until the person experiences something that he interprets as possibly indicating illness.

For Mr. Glover, such changes began around 10:00 in the morning. While alone at his desk he began to experience general unease and discomfort and, then, during the next few minutes, growing "pressure" over his mid-anterior chest and an aching sensation down the left arm to the elbow. The similarity of these symptoms to those of his previous heart attack quickly came to his mind. Thus began the threat of disruption at the *person* level and with it another wave of reverberations up and down the systems hierarchy.

The role played by the central nervous system now became critical, first in the integration and regulation of his inner experiences and his behavioral responses and second in the physiological adjustments that were occurring in response to the processes in the oxygen-deprived myocardium. For Mr. Glover these nervous-system-mediated processes were not in harmony. Whereas the infarcting of the myocardium called for reducing the demand for myocardial work and minimizing such arrhythmogenic factors as excessive catecholamine secretion, his psychological response was to oscillate between alarm and increased sympathetic nervous system activity on the one hand and denial and inappropriate physical activity on the other (Figure 2.3). Almost from the start, the possibility of a second heart attack came to mind, but he dismissed this in favor of "fatigue," "gas," "muscle strain," and finally "emotional tension." However, the negation itself, "*not* another heart attack," leaves no doubt that the idea of a "heart attack" was very much in his mind. Behaviorally he alternated between sitting quietly to "let it pass," pacing about the office to "work it off," and taking Alka-Seltzer.

When he could no longer deny the probability, if not the certainty, of another heart attack, a different set of concerns emerged. His new formula became, "If this really is a heart attack (but maybe it will still prove not to be), I must first get my affairs in order so that no one will be left in the lurch." In this way, he tried to sustain his self-image of competence and master and counter his fear of being helpless. But this was at the cost of imposing an even greater burden on his already overburdened heart and cardiovascular system. In systems terms, feedback was becoming increasingly positive, and a dangerous cycle was in the making. Disruptive processes at many system levels were gaining ascendancy over regulatory processes. The patient persisted in this determined, almost frenetic behavior for more than an hour, until the intervention of his employer brought it to an end and enabled him to accept hospitalization and patient status.

Figure 2.4 diagrams the psychological stabilization that took place as a result and how this led to stabilization of other systems. The intervention by the employer involved the *two-person* system, immediately affecting *person*. This terminated the vicious cycle, thereby lessening the impact on the damaged heart of potentially deleterious extra-cardiac influences.

How had the employer brought about such a felicitous result? We later learned from Mr. Glover that the employer's approach was to commend his diligence and sense of responsibility, even in the face of being so obviously ill, and to reassure him that he had left his work in suitable condition for others to take over. But she also challenged him to consider whether a higher responsibility to his family and his job did not require him to take care of himself and go to the hospital. Intuitively she had appreciated this man's need to see himself as responsible and in control, and she had sensed his deep fear of being weak and helpless. As a result, by the time Mr. Glover was admitted to the emergency department shortly before noon, he was no longer having any discomfort. The staff promptly instituted a coronary care routine. This was reassuring to the patient

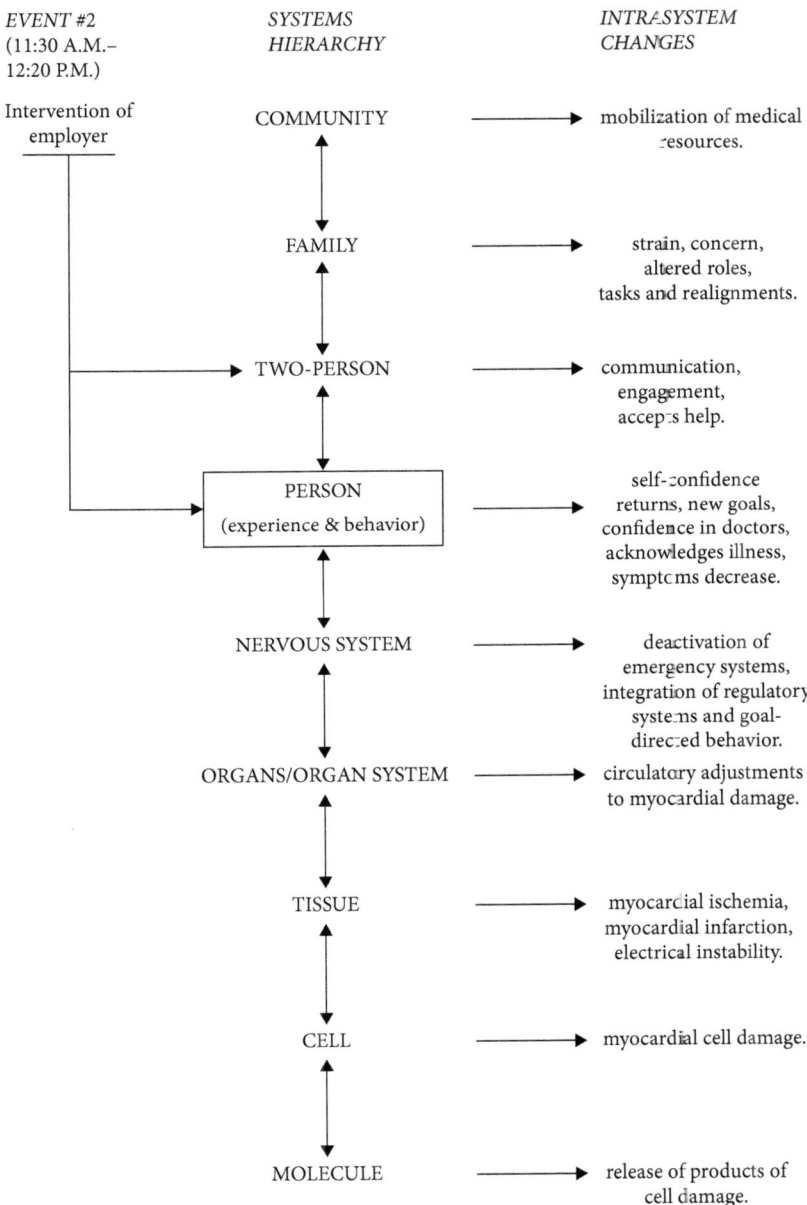

FIGURE 2.4 Biopsychosocial Model Applied

who had by now accepted the reality of a second heart attack. Thirty minutes later, in the midst of the continuing work-up, he abruptly lost consciousness. The monitor documented ventricular fibrillation. Defibrillation was successfully carried out, and the patient made an uneventful recovery.

Interviewed a few days later, Mr. Glover was able to reconstruct the events in the emergency department leading up to the cardiac arrest. His account raised doubts that the onset of ventricular fibrillation could be ascribed solely to processes originating in the injured myocardium, as the staff assumed. Rather it suggested a major role for extra-cardiac (neurogenic) influences originating in disturbances at the *two-person* and *person* levels. According to Mr. Glover, everything had been proceeding smoothly until the house officers ran into difficulty doing an arterial puncture. They persisted in their fruitless efforts for some 10 minutes and then left, explaining only that they were going for help. For Mr. Glover, the procedure was not only painful and disagreeable, but more importantly, he felt his confidence in the competence of the medical staff being undermined and with that his sense of personal mastery and control over his situation. Rather than being helped by powerful but concerned and competent professionals, he began to feel himself victimized by beginners who themselves needed help. Yet he could not bring himself to protest. His tape-recorded comment was:

> I didn't wanna tell 'em that I didn't think, ah, that I knew, he wasn't doing it right ... they tried here and they tried there ... the poor fellow was having such a tough time, he just couldn't get it.

Within a short time, the patient found himself getting hot and flushed. Chest pain recurred and quickly became as severe as it had been earlier that morning. When the staff left to get help, he first felt relieved. However, anticipating more of the same, he began to feel outrage and then to blame himself for having permitted himself to be trapped in such a predicament. A growing sense of impotence to do anything about his situation culminated in his passing out as ventricular fibrillation supervened.

## THE TWO MODELS COMPARED

Figure 2.5 diagrams the unsuccessful attempt at arterial puncture. It provides an opportunity to draw a contrast between how the model that organizes a physician's thinking also influences the physician's approach. In the case of Mr. Glover, the judgment to institute an acute coronary regimen without delay is beyond dispute. Where differences emerge are in the priorities set and the behavior displayed by adherents of each model as they go about their study and care of the patient. The emergency room approach was conventionally and narrowly biomedical. It was predicated on the reductionist premise that the cause of Mr. Glover's problem, and therefore the requirements for this care, could be localized to the myocardial injury. Because of that assumption, plus the high risk attendant on such injury, they felt justified proceeding with the technical diagnostic and treatment procedures and gave only passing attention to how Mr. Glover was feeling and reacting. When the arrest occurred, the staff congratulated each other and the patient on his good fortune, pointing out that had his arrival in the hospital been delayed another 30 minutes, he might well not have survived. They assumed that the onset of ventricular fibrillation at 12:30 p.m. could be ascribed solely to the natural progression of the myocardial injury.

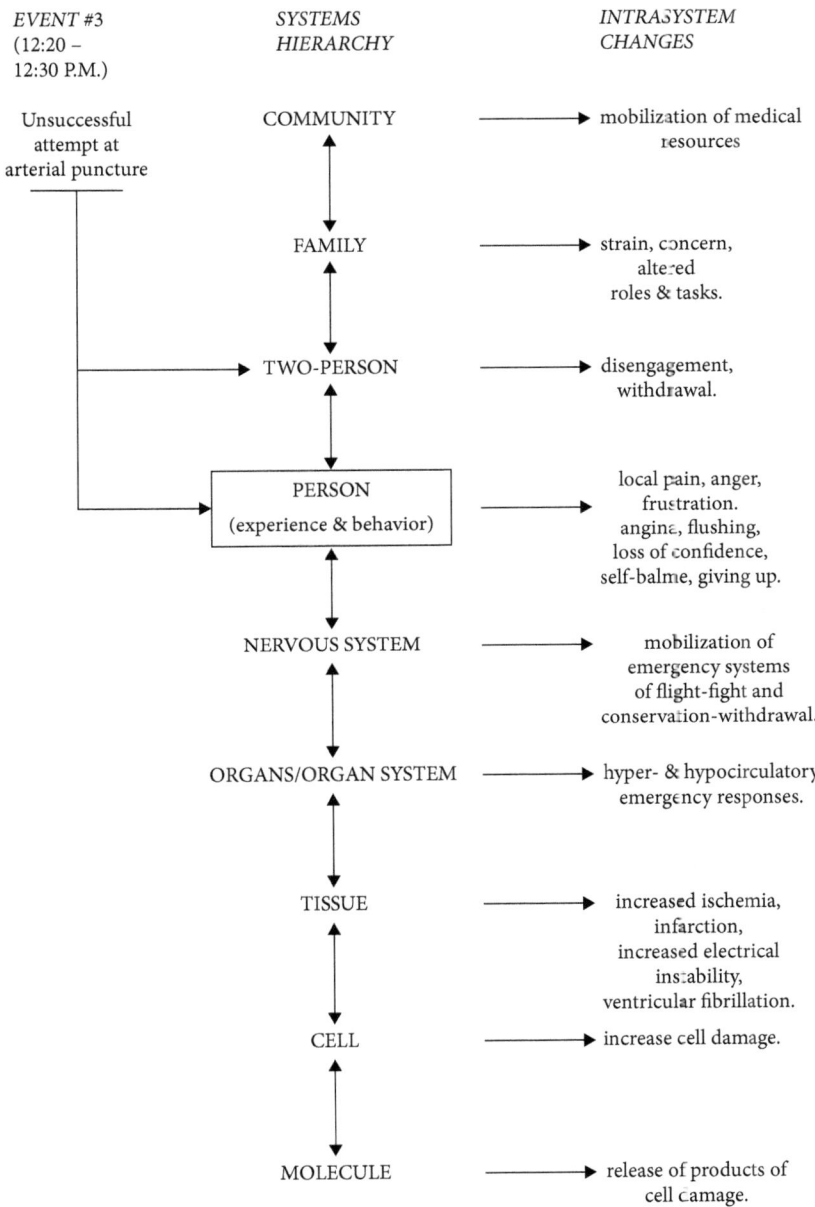

FIGURE 2.5 The Two Models Compared

A systems approach to Mr. Glover would have differed in notable respects. From the outset, the decision for the implementation of coronary care would have included consideration of factors other than cardiac status, notably those manifest at the *person* level. The initial interview of Mr. Glover would have been conducted so as to elicit simultaneously information needed to characterize him as a person as well as to evaluate the status of his cardiovascular system. Particularly in the case of a possible myocardial infarction, the systems-oriented physician would be alert to information about *person*-level factors that might alter the stability of the cardiovascular system. For example, to learn how the employer had helped him accept the reality of his heart attack and the need for prompt medical attention would be considered helpful in guiding the physician's approach to the patient. Moreover, as the coronary care regimen was being implemented, the physician would also be closely monitoring the patient's reactions to the procedures. In Mr. Glover's case, this would be especially important in light of his documented reluctance to acknowledge a need for help. The difficulty with the arterial puncture would have been recognized early as a risk for the patient, not just a problem for the doctors. Mr. Glover's failure to complain would have been anticipated as consistent with his personality style and not interpreted as acquiescence to what was happening to him. Whether such an approach would in fact have averted the cardiac arrest is impossible to know. Certainly, sufficient experimental and clinical evidence exists linking the stress of a psychological impasse, as displayed by Mr. Glover, with increased risk of lethal arrhythmias, especially with preexisting myocardial electrical instability.

Cardiac arrest and successful defibrillation are illustrated in Figures 2.6 and 2.7, while what would have happened had resuscitation failed is diagramed in Figure 2.8. This sequence of diagrams demonstrates how higher system levels, e.g., family or community, may be affected by what is transpiring with the patient and how in turn they may then feed back to impinge on the patient with consequences for the stability of lower level systems. Indeed, sometimes the feedback from events involving the patient may contribute to morbidity, i.e., lower system destabilization, in close family members. I recently was involved in a dramatic example of such a situation.

A 59-year-old man was hospitalized on March 18 with a massive myocardial infarction. Nineteen days later his very upset wife suffered a myocardial infarction while visiting her husband. For several days she had been having chest pains which she kept to herself lest she upset her husband. The latter had been recuperating and was to be discharged April 6, but early that morning he was found dead. His wife, who had anticipated his visit at 9:00 a.m. before he went home, died suddenly when she learned why he was not coming. Her final words were, "Oh, no, no, Doctor, why did it happen?" and then, "Oh, no, I'm going, too." She died of a ruptured ventricle.

Some argue that the biopsychosocial model imposes an impossible demand on the physician. That misses the point. The model does not add anything to what is not already involved in patient care. Rather, it provides a conceptual framework and encourages a way of thinking that enables the physician to act rationally in areas until now excluded from a rational approach. Furthermore, it motivates the physician to become more informed and skillful in the psychosocial areas, disciplines now seen as alien and remote even by those who intuitively recognize their importance. The biopsychosocial physician is expected to have a working knowledge of the principles, language, and basic facts of each relevant discipline; he is not expected to be an expert at all.

The example of Mr. Glover, despite its oversimplification, indicates how the working conceptual model the physician uses can influence the approach to patient care.

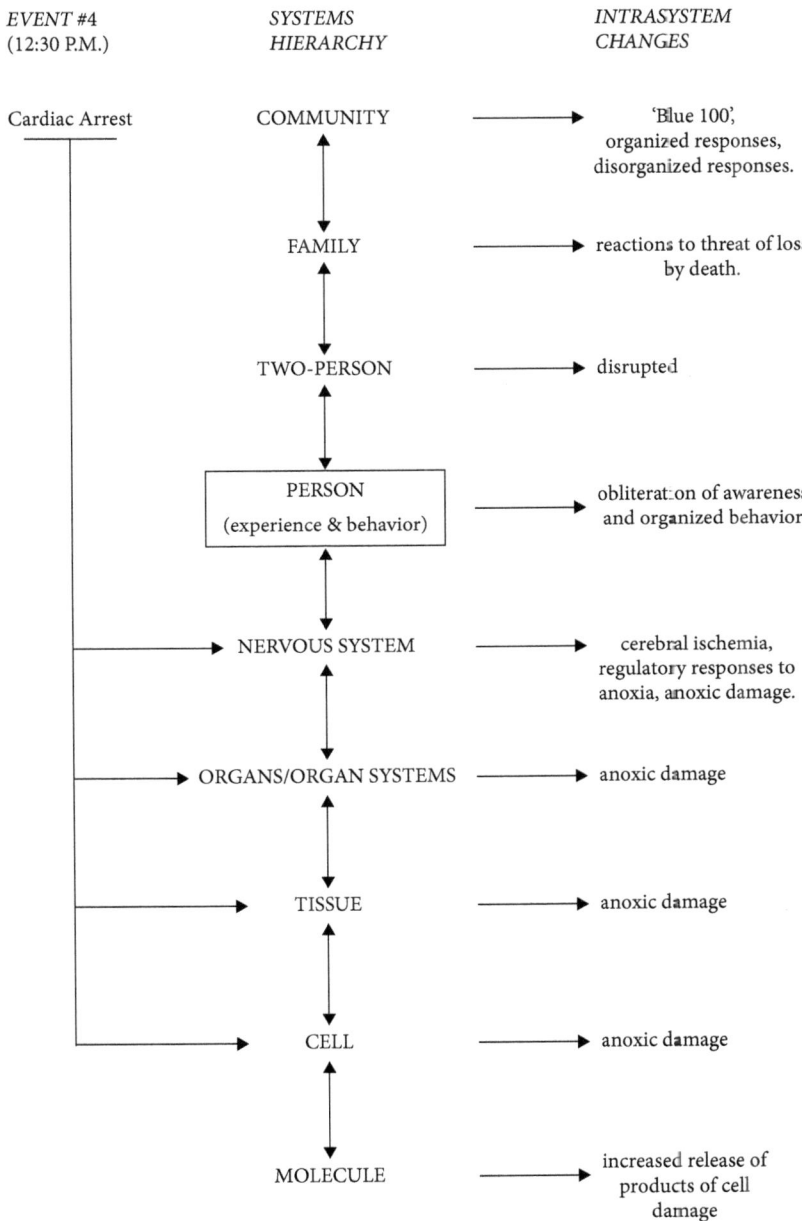

FIGURE 2.6 The Two Models Compared

The biopsychosocial model is a scientific model. The biomedical model evolved as a scientific model, but by now it has become transformed into a folk model, actually the dominant folk model of the Western world. As such, it has come to constitute dogma. The hallmark of a scientific model is that it provides a framework within which the scientific method may be applied. The value of a scientific model is measured not by

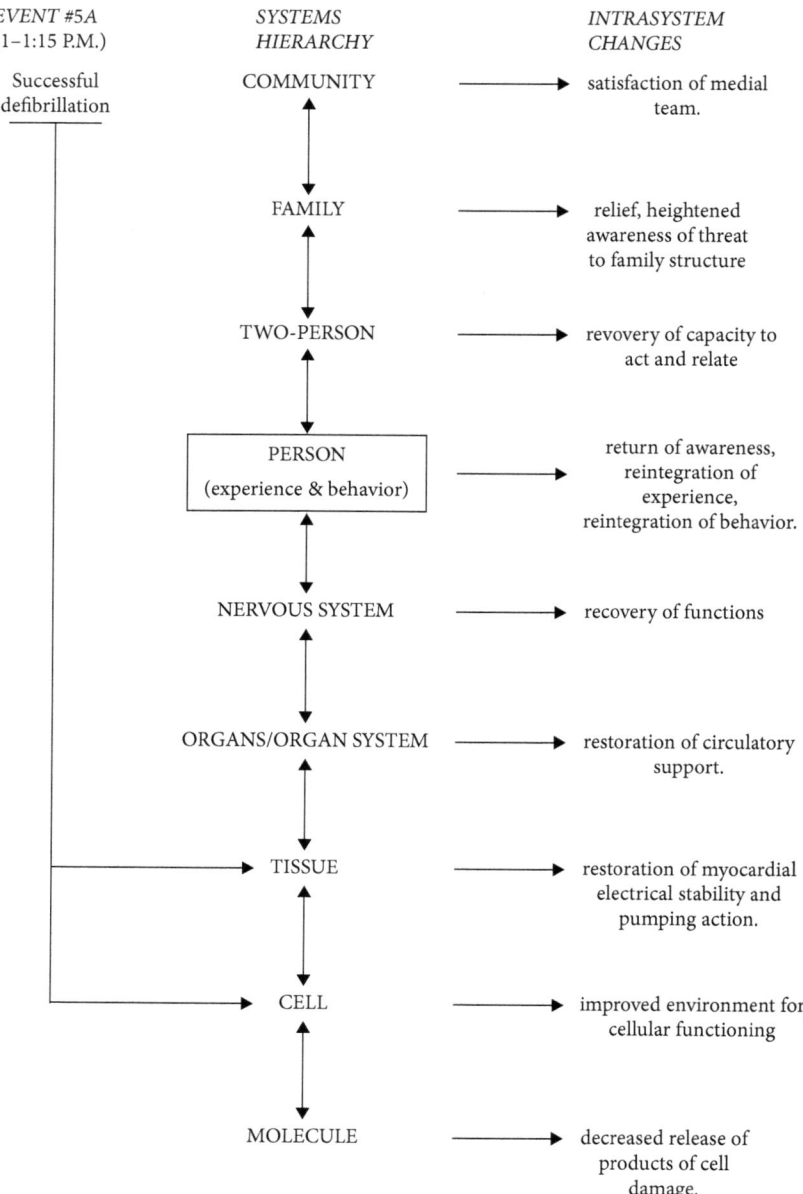

FIGURE 2.7 The Two Models Compared

whether it is right or wrong but by how useful it is. It is modified or discarded when it no longer helps to generate and test new knowledge. Dogmas, in contrast, maintain their influence through authority and tradition. They resist change and hence tend to promote opposition and the promulgation of rival dogmas by dissident figures. The counter-dogmas being put forth these days in opposition to biomedical dogma are

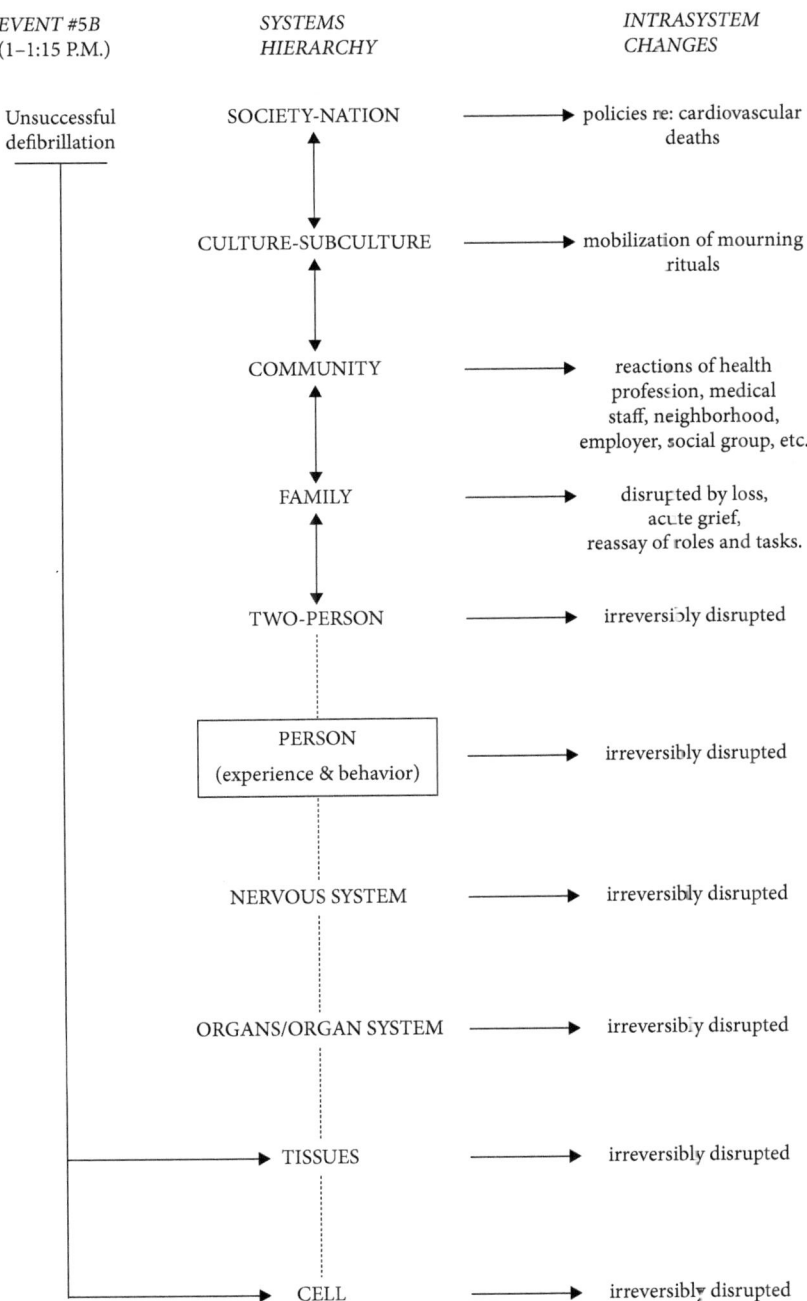

FIGURE 2.8 The Two Models Compared

sometimes called "holistic" and "humanistic" medicine. They qualify as dogmas to the extent that they often eschew the scientific method and lean instead on faith and belief systems handed down from remote and obscure or charismatic authority figures. They tend to place science and humanism in opposition. However, as the history of the biomedical model itself has shown, progress is made only where the scientific method is applied. The triumphs of the biomedical model all have been in the areas for which the model has provided a suitable framework for scientific study. The biopsychosocial model extends that scientific framework to heretofore neglected areas.

## SUGGESTED READINGS

Engel, G. L. 1971. Sudden and rapid death during psychological stress: Folklore or folkwisdom? Ann. Intern. Med. 74: 771–782.

Engel, G. L. 1977. The need for a new medical model: A challenge for biomedicine. Science 196: 129–136.

Peabody, F. W. 1927. The care of the patient. JAMA 88: 877–882.

Von Bertalanffy, L. 1968. General System Theory. Braziller, New York.

Weiss, P. 1967. 1 + 1 = 2: When one plus one does not equal two. In: G. C. Quarton, T. Melnechuk, and F. O. Schmidt (eds): The Neurosciences: A Study Program, pp. 801–821. Rockefeller Univ. Press, New York.

Weiss, P. 1977. The system of nature and the nature of systems: empirical holism and practical reductionism harmonized. In: K. E. Schaefer, K. E. Hensel, and R. Bordy (eds): Towards a Man-Centered Medicine Science, pp. 17–64. Futura, Mt. Kisco, New York.

# 3

# CARE OF THE PATIENT: ART OR SCIENCE?

*George L. Engel*

For centuries medicine has stubbornly clung to the view that the study of disease is a science while the care of the patient is an art. Because art is believed to be more dependent on personal qualities than on principles that can be examined and communicated, it is widely accepted that the art of medicine cannot be taught: At best it can be demonstrated only by precept and example. This dichotomous view that restricts science to disease while relegating the care of the patient to the "mystic" realm of art is the basis for the frequently voiced complaint that physicians have become too scientific and not sufficiently concerned with patients as human beings. Such complaints have been heard for more than 150 years. From time to time, however, a few have questioned if the reverse is not the case—if medicine's neglect of a scientific approach to its human side does not in fact mean that medicine has not yet become scientific enough.

In this chapter, I put forth the thesis that the care of the patient is as much a matter for science as is the study of disease, and that both involve art and require artistry as well. Behavior, feelings, human transactions, and relationships—and hence patient care—are indeed amenable to examination and study through application of the scientific method. It is possible to make precise observations of human behavior and to describe them verbally, to characterize and classify psychosocial data, to establish reliability, to draw inferences, and to develop testable hypotheses. It *is* possible to establish generalizations about patient care that have predictive value and provide reliable guides for how the physician should behave under particular circumstances. Once derived, such principles *can* be communicated, tested, refined, and applied by others.

Let us first specify that patient care encompasses all of the interpersonal and social transactions between the patient and the various health providers; it is not the responsibility of the physician alone, though this discussion is limited to the role of the physician. In practical terms, decisions concerning a patient's care are being made continually by the physician in the course of every transaction with a patient. Implementation of such decisions is accomplished through the doctor's behavior, by what is said or done—as well as by what is not said or done—and how it is or is not said or done. The ultimate goal of a scientific approach to patient care is that the basis for the decisions and the means of their implementation be rendered consciously rational and accessible to reporting. Decisions must not be personally idiosyncratic, mysteriously intuitive, or professionally ritualized—too often the manner in which physicians do make patient care decisions. They must be predicated on reliable data correctly interpreted and on principles amenable to scientific study and validation. Such standards must apply as much to minute-to-minute micro decisions as to more major decisions, e.g., whether to linger a moment longer at the bedside as well as when and how to propose open-heart surgery.

In the treatment of disease, the time-honored precept has been: "Assist Nature and do no needless harm." For patient care a corresponding precept might be: "Assist Human Nature and provoke no needless upset." The doctor's task is to identify the patient's psychological strengths and social resources and help him make the best use of them. At the same time, the doctor must also provide the emotional and practical support needed to help compensate for existing weaknesses and deficits. The decisions made and the actions taken by the physician must as much as possible maximize confidence, hope, and equanimity and minimize needless emotional upset or social disruption.

To illustrate how Human Nature may be hindered, not assisted, and the patient unnecessarily upset, let us turn to an actual incident. From this we may consider how the outcome may have been different had the doctor involved based his decision and behavior on a scientific understanding of human nature.

A middle-aged woman with a history of intermittent drinking and fatty liver had been abstemious for several years. She had been feeling relatively well until 6 weeks before admission when anorexia, fatigability, weakness, and loss of pep and interest abruptly developed. Her physician concurred with her concern that perhaps her liver trouble had flared up; he admitted her to the hospital for liver studies, including biopsy.

All the laboratory findings proved unremarkable, and her doctor was now coming to report the results of the biopsy. As a visitor I was accompanying my host on his morning rounds. Approaching the bedside together, he gave me a thumbnail sketch of the case, adding: "I am sure she will be glad to know the outcome of the liver biopsy." He greeted her with a cheerful smile and wave of his hand saying, "Good news, Mrs. Jones, the biopsy shows only a *little* fat in the liver, so you can leave the hospital in the morning. I'm sure you'll be glad to get home to your family."

The patient smiled faintly but said nothing as the doctor began efficiently to palpate her abdomen while asking, "And how *are* you today?" After momentary hesitation she responded rather wanly, "Pretty good, I guess," at the same time frowning slightly and raising, then letting fall, her right hand in a gesture of helplessness.

"Good," said the doctor, "I'm glad to hear that," and walked out of the room with a smile.

The patient looked so disconsolate that I lingered behind, commenting, "You don't seem so happy about this." She burst into tears. Encouraged by my interest, she readily reported that the anorexia, fatigability, weakness, and decrease in energy had begun abruptly when she learned that her husband of 25 years was leaving her for another woman. She acknowledged feeling rejected and hurt but denied that she had resumed drinking. She had hoped to be able to share this information with her doctor, but she claimed, he gave her no opportunity. When I subsequently inquired of him, he expressed surprise at the information and amazement at how readily she had revealed it to me.

Our discussion here is limited to the decisions that bear on patient-care, which the doctor made during the few minutes at the bedside. As must be clear, they were predicated on both faulty information and poor observation. Indeed, they reflected more the physician's own needs and a ritualized pattern of behavior than they did a response to the patient's situation at the moment. The basic requirements of a scientific approach were ignored, presumably because the physician's education had not allowed him to appreciate that such was possible. We can be confident that his intentions were of the best—to make the patient feel better—and that he would no more knowingly and needlessly upset his patient than he would administer a drug contraindicated in liver disease. He was a clinician whose standards would not permit him to make decisions about the treatment of the liver disease without first establishing the pertinent facts. Yet he made decisions about her life without first investigating her current life situation and emotional status. Furthermore, he persisted in his decision in the face of a clear sign from the patient, the hesitant response and the gesture of helplessness, indicating that he had overlooked something. Such behavior on the part of the physician is equivalent to persisting in the administration of a drug contraindicated in liver disease in the face of jaundice and a palpable liver.

What, you may ask, does this have to do with science? Is this not merely an example of a physician singularly lacking in sensitivity, judgment, and common sense? (He was in fact a distinguished clinical teacher and investigator, greatly admired by his peers and his students.) The question may perhaps be answered best by reviewing how the scientific method was utilized to establish the meaning of the sign that the doctor had overlooked, i.e., the gesture that indicates a feeling of helplessness. By so doing, I hope to document that clinically relevant psychological phenomena are indeed amenable to scientific study.

## SCIENTIFIC READING OF NONVERBAL LANGUAGE

First, let us describe the gesture more fully: It is typically biphasic. When fully developed, both hands are raised fairly briskly to the level of the face, the elbows flexed, the palms facing each other and rotated slightly outward, the fingers spread, and the thumb and fingers slightly flexed as though preparing to grasp. This position is held for a second or less and then the hands fall limply with gravity. Abortive and incomplete gestures may also be seen. Thus the hands may be raised through only part of the arc, or only one hand may be lifted a few inches, rotated outward with fingers spread and then allowed to fall back. Sometimes the upward movement of the hands is accompanied by an upward glance, a slight elevation of the brow and lid, and a slight tilt backward of the head. As hands fall, the face may sag and the body slump as well.

Certainly this gesture must be familiar to all of you, but whether you consciously associate it with a feeling of helplessness, or even understand helplessness as an affect, is another matter. This is because non-verbal expressions of affects, e.g. gestures, postures, facial expressions, and tone of voice, evoke feelings more often than they stimulate a conscious intellectual response. Hence although we may differ in how sensitive we are to the emotional expressions of others, by and large most of us "feel" before we "know" what the other person is experiencing and communicating. Furthermore, we typically respond to and act on such feelings, at least initially, more in terms of our own emotional needs of the moment than in terms of the other person's situation. Thus a non-verbal expression that is threatening (e.g., anger) or demanding (e.g., helplessness or anxiety) may elicit overreaction or even be screened out altogether lest our own equanimity be threatened. As physicians committed to helping others in distress, however, we must go beyond our own feelings to understand what the patient is feeling and trying to communicate. This can be achieved through developing a scientific typology of gestures, postures, and facial expressions and establishing their relationship to the inner experiences being felt and expressed. Armed with such knowledge, a physician can regard such communications more objectively as signs as well as experience them empathically as feelings. How has this been accomplished with respect to the feeling of helplessness?

Schmale, in the course of his studies of psychological giving up, first formulated the concept of helplessness as an affect. Put into words, helplessness means, "I give up, there is nothing further I can do, no way I can cope by myself; only someone else or altered circumstances can help." Developmentally, Schmale relates the feeling of helplessness to that period from birth to 2 to 3 years when the child is totally or largely dependent on adults for even its most elementary needs.

The proof of the association between the gesture and the feeling derives from the following sources:

1. Verbal expression of helplessness and giving up often is accompanied by the gesture.
2. A familiar metaphor to express the inability to do anything further upon encountering a perceived impasse is "to throw up one's hands."
3. Volunteers directed under hypnosis to display through bodily expression the feeling of helplessness characteristically exhibited the gesture. They did not do so in response to the suggestion of 13 other affects.
4. For the small child, to be held in the parent's arms means comfort, security, and protection. When in distress, toddlers characteristically communicate their need for help by looking up and raising the hands, i.e., by signaling a wish to be picked up and held. This corresponds to the first phase of the helplessness gesture. Frame-by-frame analysis of motion pictures documents that the position of the upraised hands is the same as that of the toddler asking to be picked up. Thus to look up and to raise the hands are behaviors learned early in life to signal a need for help.
5. When active efforts to adjust to a changing environment prove to no avail, life may be preserved by withdrawal, inactivity, and disengagement, a biological regulatory process we have termed *conservation–withdrawal*. We suggest that the muscular hypotonia characterizing this process in primates accounts for the falling of arms with gravity that marks the second phase of the helplessness gesture.

Thus the helplessness gesture begins with the bodily communication of a wish to be picked up, only to be superseded by the hypotonia of conservation-withdrawal, as the very reaching for help emphasizes its futility at the moment. In the process, the need for help is communicated. The gesture is embedded in both the developmental biology of the infant–adult relationship and the biological regulatory processes of conservation–withdrawal. As far as we have been able to learn, it is a universal gesture.

Let us now turn to the clinical example that stimulated this discussion. I leave it to you to decide if the elucidation of the meaning of the gesture constitutes proper application of the scientific method. If you agree, then you must also agree that the doctor's failure to recognize and respond appropriately to the gesture was no more consistent with scientific medicine than would have been his failure to detect and respond appropriately to an enlarged liver. In this instance, the helplessness gesture not only indicated the unreliability of the patient's verbal response, "Pretty good, I guess," it also provided the physician with a second opportunity to consider another diagnosis, i.e., that the patient was feeling depressed. In light of this woman's propensity to resort to alcohol under such circumstances, his failure to correctly interpret and respond to his patient's behavior in fact placed her already damaged liver at greater risk. Clearly, to have assisted Human Nature here would also have assisted Nature.

Let us consider another example. The experienced scientific clinician, familiar with basic pathophysiological principles and how such processes are manifested in clinical terms, is often remarkably successful in drawing correct inferences from a relatively limited set of observations. This is because experience has documented for him a high probability that certain clinical phenomena relate to each other and in turn correlate with particular underlying pathophysiological processes. For example, when a clinician sees a patient propped up with pillows and gasping for breath, he immediately thinks of congestive heart failure. This constitutes a hypothesis, the correctness of which can quickly be tested by further history and examination. The ability to draw such high level inferences from relatively limited data and to know how to test them is indispensable for the successful identification and correct treatment of disease. The scientific physician is able at a glance to recognize cardinal manifestations, to derive from them plausible hypotheses, and to devise appropriate means to test such hypotheses. As a scientist, he is meticulous about the reliability and relevance of the methods he uses, diligent in verifying the validity of the data, and attentive to alternative hypotheses before he resolves on a course of action. Such commitment to the scientific method is by no means incompatible with the fact that clinical circumstances sometimes require the physician to make decisions and to act before all the facts are known or all the relevant hypotheses have been formulated and tested. Conscientious adherence to the scientific method is what differentiates the competent physician from the hack and the quack.

These principles are well recognized and observed in the diagnosis and treatment of disease. Do they not apply equally for the understanding and care of the patient? They do indeed, and it is only the widely held assumption that such matters are not amenable to a scientific approach that has prevented their inclusion in the education of medical students. Let me illustrate with an example of how bits of behavior may also justify drawing inferences pertinent to the care of the patient and how in turn the validity of such inferences can be tested.

While serving as visiting professor of medicine at another institution, I was asked at grand rounds to interview a man who 9 days earlier had suffered a cardiac arrest and been successfully resuscitated. The only information made available to me was that he was a retired businessman of 64 whose arrest had occurred in the parking lot of the hospital. Let us call him Mr. John.

The amphitheater was crowded, and there was barely enough room for the two of us when Mr. John, a somewhat portly, gray-haired, well-groomed man was wheeled in. In quick succession, the patient exhibited three telling bits of behavior. First, in a rapid yet nonetheless deliberate manner, he carefully scanned the auditorium, his expression changing from a slightly quizzical frown to a faint smile in the few seconds this took. Then apparently he noticed there was not room enough for both his wheelchair and my chair. As the house officer was attempting to maneuver the wheelchair into place and before I had even sized up what the difficulty was, the patient from his wheelchair began to move my chair. He ended up directing me and the resident until the two chairs were located to his satisfaction.

As the interview began I was holding a hand microphone which after my initial question I extended toward him for his response. Then came the third bit of behavior. Mr. John at once took the microphone from my hand and responded, gazing alternately from me to the audience. Thereafter it was he, not I, who controlled the microphone. When he had finished saying what he had to say, and only then, did he direct the microphone toward me for my next question.

What inferences, if any, may one draw from such a small sample? As with the example of the orthopneic patient referred to earlier, the answer depends on one's fund of knowledge, grasp of basic principles, and ability to make reliable observations—this time, however, in the realm of human behavior rather than pathophysiology. Few, I suspect, would disagree that this patient's behavior constituted an effort on his part to establish and maintain control in a new situation. However, such a formulation is a mere tautology, comparable to stating that our orthopneic patient was trying to get more air into his lungs.

Our scientific approach demands that we look much further. This patient's behavior, it seemed to me, was all the more remarkable considering the fact that it was displayed a mere 9 days after a cardiac arrest. Subdued, passive behavior might seem more plausible under such circumstances. Actually, this patient's behavior during the first minute of the interview immediately brings to mind the behavior and personality characteristics that many investigators, beginning with Osler in 1896, have reported among patients who develop coronary artery and cerebrovascular disease. Friedman and Roseman popularized this pattern as Type A.

For a physician to make such a generalization on the basis of merely one minute of observation is no different than would be his thinking of congestive heart failure and its pathogenesis upon observing a propped-up patient gasping for breath. In both examples the generalization also predetermines the questions to be asked and the strategies to be invoked to test its validity for the patient in question. In this case, we first needed to establish whether this behavior constituted a specific reaction to the situation of being presented at rounds or reflected a more enduring personality style. A mere 15 minutes of interviewing supported the latter. As Mr. John spoke about his hospital experience, the circumstances of his illness, his business career, his personal relationships and family life, his satisfactions and frustrations, and his life style, item after item emerged consistent with Type A personality. His personal account of himself and his life, comprised of incidents, experiences, relationships, and expressions of opinion, judgments, and self-characterizations, added up to the picture of an aggressive, ambitious man, always active, busy and planning, and preoccupied with deadlines, high standards of performance, and self-set goals; a man who basically felt he could depend only on himself to get the job done and to [ensure] gratification of his own needs. To a remarkable degree, his behavior upon entertaining the amphitheater accurately reflected many of these characteristics.

On the basis of our knowledge of psychological settings that seem especially conducive to sudden death, we entertained a second hypothesis. Experience has shown that the risk of cardiac arrest in the biologically vulnerable Type A person is greatest when the patient feels or actually is in danger of losing his sense of control over his environment, the more so if preceded by a period of discouragement and depression or accompanied by strong feelings of fear, anger, or excitement that culminate in a sense of futility or failure. In the case of this 64-year-old man, we learned that the patient's carefully laid plans to devote his retirement to "doing his own thing" had been thwarted by his daughter's divorcing and leaving the care of her 3- and 4-year-old children to Mr. John and his wife. To make matters worse, the older boy had then become ill. Rather than playing golf and cultivating his many new hobbies, Mr. John now felt burdened with these unwanted responsibilities as well as disappointed in his daughter. The cardiac arrest occurred on the way to the doctor's office with the 4-year-old when a parking space for which he had been patiently waiting was "stolen" by another motorist. He remembers angrily shaking his fist at the motorist, driving off, and nothing more. In the interview he described this episode as "the last straw." An acute myocardial infarction 5 years earlier placed him in the group at higher risk for cardiac arrest.

## BIOPSYCHOSOCIAL MODEL AS BASIS FOR TREATMENT STRATEGIES

Perhaps you concede that this is interesting, maybe even persuasive, but the more skeptical among you may still be wondering how such information contributes to more effective patient care, in this case care of the Type A patient. The answer to that question requires a further step. If we are to assist Human Nature, as we earlier defined the goal of patient care, then we must know what these psychological characteristics, so readily established through proper observational and interview techniques, mean for the patient. Understanding this, we can also infer how the physician's approach to the patient may be adapted to minimize distress and encourage confidence and peace of mind. Scientifically, this requires a different level of conceptualization and a different strategy of investigation. It corresponds to *explaining* orthopnea rather than merely *recognizing* it as a cardinal manifestation of left ventricular failure. For orthopnea this requires elucidating the underlying pathophysiology; for Type A behavior it requires elucidating the underlying psychodynamics.

Basic knowledge of psychodynamics, like basic knowledge of pathophysiology, is best achieved through long-term or in-depth study of a few patients. Among persons exhibiting Type A behavior, a variety of unconscious determinants have been uncovered, the most critical of which is a deep-seated fear of being put in a passive, helpless, or dependent position. Typical Type A individuals exaggerate the opposite traits, striving always to be active, independent, and in control of the environment and the people in it. In the process they become their own most severe critics and exacting taskmasters. They continually set and then strive to fulfill higher and higher goals for themselves and others, thereby repetitively subjecting themselves to the risk of failure, a failure for which they characteristically take personal responsibility. By the same token, the deep fear of helplessness and passivity also makes it difficult for them to rest on their laurels; no matter how successful, they must constantly strive after more success, a situation both encouraged and aggravated by societies that place a high premium on performance and achievement, as does our Western industrialized society. Suffice it to say, the physician's failure to take into account these underlying dynamics may have serious consequences for the patient, as the example of Mr. Glover in Chapter 2 illustrates.

Psychologically speaking, the circumstances under which Mr. Glover's cardiac arrest occurred—the emergency department—were not all that different from those in the parking lot where Mr. John experienced a similar life-threatening attack. Would the cardiac arrest have occurred had the cardiology team in the emergency department appreciated the psychodynamics underlying the Type A personality? Indeed, would not a more knowledgeable staff have been attentive to how the patient was responding to the events in the emergency room and made a more deliberate effort to deal with his feelings before the risk of precipitating a lethal arrhythmia had reached dangerous proportions? For such a risk is very real, as clinical study and animal experiments have shown.

The answer to both of these questions must, of course, be in the affirmative. Just as an understanding of the pathophysiology of left ventricular failure enables one to appreciate the risks of recumbency, physical exertion, or excessive sodium intake, so too does understanding the psychodynamics that underlie Type A personality enable one to recognize the risks of placing such a person in a passive, helpless position, subject to the domination or control of others. Furthermore, we can readily derive from these psychodynamics rational strategies that can minimize such risks. These in turn can be tested and refined in their application, as is the case with any therapeutic measure. Let me propose, from such principles, a strategy for the care of the Type A patient with a suspected myocardial infarction.

These two patients, Mr. John and Mr. Glover, clearly illustrate that Type A personality can be suspected from the patient's reported and observed behavior during the development of the attack and from his interactions with the doctor. Once the physician is satisfied with the reasonableness of such a personality diagnosis, the challenge becomes how to take the firm command that the seriousness of the situation calls for without, at the same time, mobilizing the patient's deep-seated fear of being helpless and dominated. Obviously this is not always easy, because somehow the patient must be convinced of the doctor's command of the situation and his competence and ability to provide the help he so desperately yearns for without threatening the patient's need to continue to feel in control. This can indeed be a delicate balance, especially when the doctor also is a Type A—as many of us are—who feels threatened by patients who resist submitting to professional control. I once asked a group of medical students how they would deal with the conflict of a Type A doctor trying to take care of a Type A patient.

One proposed the following formula: In one way or another the doctor should communicate to the patient, "All my skills and all my knowledge are at your command." An elegant compromise! For thereby each preserves relative autonomy. For the patient it facilitates the illusion that he commands the doctor, while at the same time communicating the reality that it is the doctor (and surrogates) who is the sole possessor of the critical knowledge and skills.

In practice, care of the Type A patient requires monitoring of psychological processes, undertaken as carefully as one monitors cardiac rhythm on the EKG to assess the patient's continuing struggle to maintain autonomy while submitting to the demands of the treatment. The very fact of the doctor's interest in the coronary patient's concerns over such issues, however expressed, can itself powerfully contribute to a growing sense of trust on the part of the patient, something not easily achieved by individuals with Type A personality traits. At the same time, the patient's awareness that the doctor is interested in and wants to understand whatever may be contributing to the patient's concerns enables the patient to feel progressively more relaxed in relinquishing some of his own needs to maintain control. Accordingly, judicious interventions (e.g., providing the patient with access to a phone or to a visitor, even in the Emergency Department, so that unfinished business can be resolved) may both relieve the patient's anxiety as well as provide assurance that he has not been capriciously stripped of all his command. Helpful too are trade-offs, the concession of lesser activities in place of more taxing ones, especially when done in such a way that the patient is given the feeing of participating in the decision to relinquish one activity in favor of another. The interactions between physician and patient, in the course of which information and concerns are shared and decisions agreed on, provide the matrix in which the patient eventually succeeds in identifying with the powerful doctor, thereby symbolically acquiring the doctor's strengths and sense of competence. In this way, the physician comes to be seen as a helpful surrogate rather than as a menacing adversary. The patient who says, "I discussed this with my doctor and *we decided* . . ." often is expressing such a successful identification.

The care of the patient, no less than the treatment of organ-level disease processes is a matter for science; excellence in both reflects the art with which the physician applies scientific knowledge. The power of dogma is great. More than a hundred years ago, Sir William Gull warned against the dogmatism of a too physiochemically oriented "Science, by throwing the light of particular inquiry full in our eyes, blinds us for a time to that which lies beyond." The remarkable accomplishments of biomedical research and technology have had just such an unforeseen side effect. The challenge now is to expand our horizons and at long last begin to apply the scientific method with the same vigor to the understanding of human feelings and behavior as we have to the understanding of disease and pathophysiology. Enhancement of patient care and human well-being cannot help but follow.

## SUGGESTED READINGS

Engel, G. L. 1971. Sudden and rapid death during psychological stress: Folklore or folkwisdom? Ann. Intern. Med. 74: 771–782.

Engel, G. L. 1974. Signs of giving up. In: S. B. Troup and W. A. Greene (eds): The Patient, Death, and the Family, pp. 45–72. Charles Scribner, New York.

Engel, G. L., and Schmale, A. H. 1972. Conservation-withdrawal: a primary regulatory process for organismic homeostasis. In: R. Porter and J. Knight (eds): Physiology, Emotion and Psychosomatic Illness, pp. 57–85. Ciba Foundation Symposium 8 (New Series). Elsevier-Excerpta Medica, Amsterdam.

Friedman, M. 1969. Pathogenesis of Coronary Artery Disease, pp. 78–104. McGraw-Hill, New York.

Gull, W. W. 1976. Clinical observation in relation to medicine in modern times. In: T. D. Acland (ed): Collection of the Published Writings of William Withey Gull. Memoirs and Addresses, p. 38. The New Sydenham Society, London.

Schmale, A. H. 1962. Needs, gratifications and the vicissitudes of the self-representation: a developmental concept of psychic: object relationships. Psychoanal. Stud. Soc. 2: 9–41.

# 4

# THE DOCTOR–PATIENT RELATIONSHIP

## THE LANGUAGE OF MEDICINE

In this chapter and the one that follows, we convey to you some important notions about communicating with patients. We attempt to do so in simple English. We intend no disrespect for the often elegant, always parsimonious, and usually dispassionate language of medical science. Indeed, we were tempted to adopt a tone that was more traditional. A slew of possibilities for chapter titles came to mind—Facilitating Effective Communication Skills in the Doctor–Patient Relationship, Interviewing Skills for Health Professionals, and so on—but we refrained.

The reason we refrained has to do with the often unappreciated impact of language in the actual conduct of medicine. Let us illustrate this with a truism: The bulk of communication between doctors and patients occur in language. We "speak," of course, in many ways, but usually in words. Therefore, giving some thought to the words we doctors and patients use to talk to each other may not be entirely trivial. Consider the doctor–patient relationship by means of simple analogy: Imagine a collaboration similar to that between a pair of mountain climbers. Their goal is to reach the top (develop an effective healing partnership). The route to the top is never entirely known in advance and requires ongoing cooperation and communication as the ascent proceeds. (The doctor–patient relationship is a process that evolves collaboratively over time.) In this analogy, we might add that one of the climbers is far more experienced in this sort of mountaineering; he has been on many similar climbs and thus often acts as an authority and guide. (The doctor has experience and expertise the patient expects, and on which the patient relies.) Still, the climbers must tackle the mountain together, and their fates are fundamentally intertwined as they make their way up a sometimes treacherous and uncharted mountain face. Finally, these two climbers—whose roles are collaborative, although not isomorphic—are bound together by critical linkages: ropes, pitons, mutually understood signals, and other means of communication. In the doctor–patient relationship, our ability to talk with each other becomes our essential arsenal of ropes and pitons. We are linked not with hemp and metal, but with words, empathy, respect, and mutual trust. To succeed, we must be able to communicate; we must be able to talk to each other and listen to each other. This is difficult at best. It becomes even more so when a person is ill, frightened, and in pain. However, it becomes impossible only if doctor and patient cannot speak the same language at all! There is no substitute for it. No CAT scan will ever be able to compensate. Thus, we are not speaking here about niceties in "the bedside manner"; we are talking about the success or failure of patient care.

How good are we doctors, then, at talking with patients? Come with us for a moment on some imaginary rounds. They are taking place in a crowded, chaotic, city hospital at 7:00 AM.

A young doctor, Dr. Miles, is trying to tell his patient that he has inoperable, metastatic cancer. Dr. Miles is white, middle class, and 27 years old. He is very committed to being the best doctor he possibly can. The patient, on the other hand, is a bit weary and worn down by life. His name is Ignacio Chavez. He is 58 years old, widowed, of Hispanic origin, and barely surviving financially on a small Medicare disability pension.

Some doctors would be able to communicate with Mr. Chavez in a meaningful way. Given the mixed degree of formal education in these skills that we provide, it is remarkable how often doctors manage to do so empathically and well. Alas, this is not so with Dr. Miles. Instead, we witness a painful series of halting stammers, equivocations, and bungled opportunities. Our young, bright doctor suddenly seems reduced to jargon and pathetic mumbles:

"You have a primary CA," he says. "There may be metastases, little pieces of it, in your vertebral column. I mean, in your spine—you know, your backbone."

Our patient, in turn, does not complain or protest. Rather, he nods and stares blankly, trying to be polite, pretending that he understands. Inside, he is also terrified, confused, and profoundly alone. These feelings emerge only later, with his family, if he is lucky enough to have a family. Or perhaps they will not come out at all. Our morning rounds end thus:

DR. MILES: Well, then, Mr. Chavez, so now you understand why I need to do the test on your spinal fluid.
MR. CHAVEZ: That's the one where you stick a needle into my back and take out some fluid?
DR. MILES: Right! It won't hurt much. Now roll over on your side and tuck up your knees to your chin.
MR. CHAVEZ: (No verbal response, silently assumes position as instructed.)

Our young doctor performs the lumbar puncture, collects the samples, and places a small Band-Aid over Mr. Chavez's skin.

"By the way," he adds, on the way out the door, "you'll need to lie down for at least another 8 hours, and you may get a headache." Eight hours later Mr. Chavez is still lying on his bed, obedient and alone. He stares at the ceiling saying nothing. What is he thinking? It is difficult to know. His expression gives nothing away.

Is young Dr. Miles insensitive and callous? Is he hopeless? Of course not. He simply has never learned to speak with patients effectively. Not only has Dr. Miles not been trained adequately in communication skills, he has, concurrently, been socialized into a frequently dehumanized system and inculcated with biases and narrow perspectives that have actually caused a deterioration in the native compassion and empathy he originally brought with him to medical school. Like most of us, Dr. Miles went into medicine because he wanted to take care of people. What happened? The answer is complex and multifaceted. One symptom of the problem shows up in his bungling when he needs to communicate. He reverts to a highly abstruse "technical" language that confuses the patient and leaves Dr. Miles feeling more than a little uneasy. On the other hand, it is this very language that Dr. Miles knows will score points with his attending physician on rounds. Quite a predicament!

It is often said that students like Dr. Miles learn 10 000 new words in medical school. This strikes us as a conservative estimate. Yet, too often, they still cannot talk to patients and, furthermore, do not know how to listen. Certainly the problem does not lie in mastery of a very precise technical jargon. For example, students learn that many anticancer agents, such as several that will be tried on Mr. Chavez, cause alopecia, ulcerative stomatitis, and desquamating intestinal enteritis. How different these words sound, if one says: These drugs may cause my patient's hair to fall out and his mouth will become filled with painful, open sores. His intestinal lining may slough off and he may bleed into his gut; the blood may come gushing out of his anus. He could bleed to death.

Despite the popular accusation, we personally do not believe doctors fall back on excessively technical language with patients to appear pretentious, smart, or to lay verbal smokescreens. More likely, the problem occurs because young doctors are not helped to cope with the emotional impact of their work. On the contrary, they are encouraged by older house officers or professors who use similar defenses to twist language so that it denies the harsh emotional realities of what patients really face and doctors really do. How could a doctor so trained then be expected to communicate effectively with a suffering patient? In truth, it is impossible to imagine an effective doctor–patient relationship emerging from an educational system that does not fully acknowledge the feelings of the doctor, let alone those of the patient.

The biopsychosocial model, which forms the central theoretical foundation of this book, is a quantum leap forward in the right direction. It yanks the feelings and relationships in a patient's life out of the clichéd realm of "bedside manner" and plants them where they should be—in the hub of scientific medicine itself. The education of future physicians must also include helping students to understand the biopsychosocial forces that they themselves experience so intensely; after all, they are half of the dyad and live in that emotionally intense crucible as surely as their patients.

One final observation about the structure of our medical language: Repeatedly, we have been struck by the propensity of all physicians to gravitate in their speech toward highly action-oriented verbs. Listen to a group of doctors talking on work rounds. They talk about "*doing* an LP." They say they need to "*get* a urine sample." They talk about "*ordering* a PA chest film." The words imply action, doing something to someone. They deny any notion of *interaction*. In one sense, this is perfectly logical. We doctors must constantly *do* things. We stick needles and cannulas into people's bodies; we withdraw fluids and tissues. Sometimes we cut bodies wide open to take out organs or even put them in. The active tone of our language thus reflects the active nature of so much of what we do. Yet, the procedures we "order" are seldom as one-sided as they at first might seem. For example, take a simple procedure: A doctor "orders" a barium enema. Yet, those of us who have observed a patient undergoing this procedure—much less endured it ourselves—appreciate how active the patient must also be. A day in advance, she is purged with harsh laxatives. She is then deprived of food. During the X-ray procedure, she must consciously squeeze her anus shut to keep a huge volume of fluids in her colon while she assumes awkward, embarrassing, and painful positions on a cold X-ray table! So the test we "ordered" is not so simple a matter as our language initially led us to think.

Imagine how different medical rounds would sound if doctors spoke like this: We need to get Mrs. Jones to our radiology technician in the morning for a really good upper GI. Or: Mr. Smith and I are going to go to the examining room at 11:00 so we can do a careful neurological; it's critical.

To some, these distinctions doubtless seem idle—the ruminations and quibbling of an obsessive lexicologist. Yet we argue the opposite. We think it is the *language* of doctors, perhaps more than any other aspect of their behavior, that betrays the difficulties they so often have dealing with powerful emotions. Over and over, physicians' choices of words reveal not only their awkwardness when they hear strong emotions in their patients, but also their limitation to seeing the doctor–patient relationship as an interaction that involves both doctor and patient (not to mention the patient's family).

## THE POWER OF THE DOCTOR–PATIENT RELATIONSHIP

A highly respected, technically gifted, humane orthopedic surgeon once made a terrible mistake. He had treated an elderly woman for many years for an arthritic condition caused by diabetes. She was very attached to him and trusted him implicitly. There came a point in her illness when the surgeon decided she would have to have her left leg operated on. She readily assented and, in due course, the operation was performed. Then, while she was in the recovery room, a tragic error was realized. The wrong leg had been draped. The surgeon had operated on the wrong knee. After considerable personal anguish, he waited for her to stabilize postoperatively and then entered her room to tell her the truth.

"Mrs. Fenswald," he began. "I have to tell you that I have made a terrible mistake. Through a series of blunders, I operated on the wrong knee."

Mrs. Fenswald initially looked shocked, then pensive. For a moment, the two sat together in silence. Then, Mrs. Fenswald replied.

"You know, Dr. Jones," she stated, "I am obviously sorry that this has happened, but I'm really not that worried. You're such a good doctor. I'm quite sure that the other knee will get better anyway."

It did!

This vignette, from Dr. Reiser's book *Patient Interviewing: The Human Dimension*,[1] is at once heartening and highly disturbing. Certainly it describes an iatrogenic catastrophe, yet it also dramatically underscores the power of the doctor–patient relationship. It is this relationship that Balint[2] has referred to as a "drug" for which "no pharmacology ... exists yet". Whatever the metaphor one chooses, and there have been many eloquent ones throughout the years, it seems indisputable that the doctor–patient relationship is one of the most powerful human dyads that exists. It is as old as history, and it exists in every culture, however "advanced" or "primitive." Despite much current lamenting about the erosion of that relationship and the demoralization that has resulted, the dyad remains, in many respects, as durable and potent as ever. If one wishes anecdotal confirmation for this, witness how often people speak in disenchanted, even enraged tones about medicine in general, yet refer in glowing terms to "my doctor." As Balint[2] points out, however, this powerful drug is not without its side effects. If the strength of the relationship can cure, it also can occasionally cause great harm, and lesser disasters occur all the time. Patients who are treated rudely and unempathically by their physician may not die from the experience, but most assuredly they will suffer. Conversely, those who feel truly understood can sometimes face great pain, uncertainty, and even death in comfort and with serenity. If one thinks about it for a moment, it is the very power of the doctor–patient relationship that explains why so many Americans are currently, and most appropriately, angry with their healers. If doctors *were* not so important, it is unlikely that people would be so disappointed and angry.

Two final points about the doctor–patient relationship deserve mention. First, neither party is ever without conflict about being part of a relationship that is so intense and important. Doctors are, understandably, ambivalent about the power invested in them and the responsibility that goes with it. Almost without exception, patients are equally ambivalent about allowing someone to be so crucially important to them. Second, although we often talk about this relationship as though it were terribly mysterious, a scientific explanation that can account for some of its incredible power is both desirable and possible. Engel's biopsychosocial approach, explicated more fully in Chapters 2 and 3, points to such an explanation. As he observes, illness almost always evokes feelings of helplessness. Such feelings can, and often do, cause patients—although they are, in fact, full-grown adults—to feel very much the way they must have felt when they were a tiny, helpless baby. Being a patient can make one feel totally dependent again, like an infant forced to rely on his parents for emotional succor and even for survival. Hence, the power of the doctor–patient relationship may derive in part from its symbolic connection to the earliest stages of life. This, of course, can be regarded only as a hypothesis, but it represents how one can use the biopsychosocial model to think scientifically about matters consigned previously to the realm of "art" and "intuition" alone. As Engel points out, people who feel that such considerations are beside the point, completely miss the point. Perhaps scientifically informed inquiries will eventually lead to the elusive pharmacology that Balint[2] laments still does not exist.

## DOCTOR–PATIENT DYAD 1: THE STUDENT AS A PERSON WITH SOMETHING TO OFFER

Medical training, from its first months to well into the house staff years, often seems diabolically contrived to make students feel they are engaged in an interminable rite of passage. They sometimes fear they are doomed to feel eternally inept, incompetent, and foolish. Students probably take little solace in reassurance that mastery and even wisdom eventually do come. For long years, medical training feels too much like a harrowing twilight of incompetence in the face of overwhelming responsibilities and stress to permit students any optimism about the distant, promised dawn.

Clichés do not mollify students on this point. It is often more helpful to suggest to these students, especially to those just beginning, that they actually have something to offer their patients.

## A Biopsychosocial Perspective

To begin with, and at the very least, students can offer their unbiased presence. There is some irony here. Very often, precisely because students have not yet grown excessively encumbered and narrowed by an exclusively biomedical viewpoint, they can actually interact with patients in some important and therapeutic ways that may be overlooked by their more medically jaded mentors. Students often dismiss this advantage as mere naiveté, "being a nice person"—the bone students toss to patients in view of being able to do anything "real" for them. All this, they complain, is accompanied by the "fraudulent" donning of the white coat, and what at times feels like the endless exploitation of patients as "guinea pigs." Reassurance alone does little to assuage most students' anxieties about these matters.

In fact, however, students are in an ideal position to approach patients from the perspective of the biopsychosocial model. Ironically, students may be the most free to see their patients as parts of a total system—from mitochondria to ministers, from white blood cells to wives. The students' relative freedom to learn and apply the biopsychosocial model to patient care can be an invaluable asset. This is one important reason why students, despite their relative technical inexperience, so often form relationships of such tremendous richness with their patients.

## Curiosity

Students are usually curious. They are curious about the body and the mind, and about the ways in which the two interact. Although they fear asking something "dumb" on rounds, students in fact are encumbered by far fewer stereotypes than their mentors. Furthermore, their curiosity can be channeled and trained. With guidance, it can be honed from diffuse fascination to an astute capacity for accurate and detailed observation. The great diagnostic value of such observational skills is discussed more fully in the next chapter.

## Compassion

Students occasionally find themselves mocked for their compassion by only slightly older peers. More egregious, perhaps, is the widespread folklore that depicts medical students as cut-throat, narrow-minded, and compulsive—survivors of the "dog eat dog" competitive system of premedical training that got them into medical school. Actually, nothing could be less true. Students rarely begin as the ruthless, conniving gunners they are sometimes made out to be. If they finally end up that way, it is because they are made to fit that caricature by powerful, even irresistible pressures for social conformity that beset them during their medical training. Medical schools are inundated with so many qualified applicants; it would behoove them to admit the intellectually superior, morally outstanding, and deeply sensitive male and female applicants.

Students can and frequently do bring a capacity for concern and compassion to their patients. It is vital to a patient's well-being. This is one of the ironic reasons patients, especially at training hospitals, so often refer to the medical student assigned to them as "my real doctor." One student, for example, had this experience when he was still a freshman. He was working with a middle-aged woman who was dying of cancer. At a certain point, surgical removal of her ovaries seemed desirable as a palliative measure. The woman refused. Finally, the chairman of the department of surgery attempted to prevail on her.

"Not until you get permission from my doctor!" she insisted. Ultimately, there was the whimsical spectacle of a prominent surgery professor being given "permission" by a freshman medical student to perform the operation. The incident cuts deeper than whimsy, however. In fact, this woman needed to trust in a doctor–patient relationship, and the task fell to a junior medical student bedecked in his starched, uncomfortably new, "fraudulent" white coat.

## Styles

Like patients, students have different styles. Some students are more assertive and action oriented; some, by nature, are more contemplative and slower to act. Some tend to respond on an emotional and intuitive level; others rely on logic and cognition. There is plenty of room in medicine for such a variety of styles. One of the major tasks of medical education is to assist students to learn what their own style is and to help them adapt it flexibly to a growing variety of complementary and divergent styles in their patients. Engel gives an example of this in Chapter 3, where he discusses the "Type A" physician taking care of a Type A patient. Engel's reference to Type A refers to its correlation to coronary heart disease reflective of research at the time. Research since then has shown limitations of describing complex human experiences within such narrowly defined parameters.

## Responsibility

Finally, students quickly bring to their relationships with patients something very special and important—a deep sense of responsibility. From the outset of medical training, a sense of responsibility is pounded into students. By the time they graduate, this sense has penetrated their very being. One can work at many jobs and leave the work behind at 5:00 PM when the whistle blows. Many chores and obligations can be hung like hats on pegs in a closet when the work week ends. This is not so for physicians, particularly during the training phase, when there is a felt sense that one is a physician 24 hours a day, 7 days a week, hypervigilant to digital stimuli in the environment as the pager beckons. Being a doctor is an all-consuming role that carries burdens as well as privileges, but should be contained within a structured set of duty hours to avoid the high risk of burnout and allow for nurturing of other meaningful roles within the context of personal interests, family, community, and so on.

Ironically, this deeply ingrained sense of responsibility—certainly among physicians' most noble traits—seems to be formed in part from the very same pressures in training that also promote callousness, dehumanization, and despair. To give only one example: There is no doubt that the rigorous, even brutal, on-call schedule of typical house officers, in which they are up all night every third night struggling with the suffering and pronouncing on the unquestionably dying, is a process that forges in some way the deeply internalized sense of responsibility that good physicians feel. Such a sense, of course, is not restricted to physicians, and many other individuals in other vocations also possess it. Yet, it remains one of the most important gifts medical students, even the greenest students, have to offer their patients.

## DOCTOR–PATIENT DYAD 2: THE PATIENT AS A PERSON WITH A PROBLEM

### Biopsychosocial Model

"It is more important to know what kind of patient has the disease than what kind of disease the patient has." —Sir William Osler.

A group of junior medical students and their preceptor found this out. They were conducting an interview at the bedside with a 58-year-old man who weighed 430 pounds. When the group of 7 entered the room, they found the huge man poised on the edge of the bed with almost gelatinous precariousness. Panniculus plunged pendulously to his knees. His nightshirt was mostly unbuttoned, and his pajama bottoms had slipped down below his thighs, exposing pubic hair and genitalia. Still, he beckoned the students in with a hearty laugh and showed no obvious embarrassment. His wife, a heavyset woman herself, wore thick glasses and labored at a piece of crochet work in her lap. She blushed faintly when the group entered. She had been sitting opposite her husband. Now she hurriedly pushed her chair up against the far wall, nearer to his head yet out of his line of vision. She then proceeded to watch the interview very intently but said nothing.

The student who was conducting the interview tried valiantly to ask open-ended, empathic, and appropriately leading questions—ones that would encourage the patient to open up about why he was, figuratively, eating himself to death. From the medical chart, the group knew the patient had been gaining weight since his retirement as a truck driver 10 years before. His obesity had not gotten out of hand, however, until 4 years previously, after his 24-year-old son committed suicide, leaving behind two young children. The patient mentioned none of this spontaneously. Rather, he seemed to prefer to joke cavalierly about politics and the like. Several times he said he "loved to swim." He planned to go swimming with his wife that summer, but caustically referred to her as "a hunk of blubber in the water." At one point, the wife started to interject something about the son's suicide, but he quickly cut her off. Despite the obvious drama of the events, the interview itself left a sense of boredom among the students. The patient managed to stonewall everyone. Students yawned, looked at their watches repeatedly, fidgeted, and dreamed about dinner. The preceptor stifled a yawn. When the interview finally ended 5 minutes early, all departed with a sense of relief.

The group then huddled. What had "gone wrong?" Their main data came from detailed observation and, above all, the students' ability to heed their own feelings. (This second matter is discussed further in the next chapter.) As the students conversed and conjectured, the preceptor encouraged them to delineate strictly observable data. A number of things stood out. For one, the patient seemed utterly oblivious to even the most basic amenities, apparently betraying no shame for exposing his genitals. Furthermore, he appeared mysteriously indifferent about several catastrophes in his life: his obesity, a serious urinary tract infection, and finally his son's suicide. Then there was the wife, who never said a word, except once—only to be cut off—who sat neither in nor out of the scene, vigilantly overseeing every nuance but never plunging in.

The students' ultimate formulation is discussed later in this chapter, under "Feelings." Here, simply observe that the biopsychosocial components of this man's illness were overwhelmingly obvious. This had not, incidentally, seemed so obvious before the group went to the bedside. In fact, the student who selected the patient had originally thought he only wanted the preceptor to decide whether the patient was "pickwickian"—a descriptor to describe obesity hypoventilation syndrome. He had also anticipated a discussion of the pros and cons of gastric stapling procedures in the treatment of obesity.

By the end of the interview, however, it was abundantly clear this man, with kidneys inflamed at the parenchymal level, was also shockingly emotionally disturbed. And—most troubling—he seemed to be reacting to all the tragedy with complete noblesse oblige and jocularity. Finally, this dying, infected morbidly obese man had a wife and an extended family. Somehow they had to be part of this morbid process too.

As one student exclaimed, "This man is eating himself to death! Why isn't anyone stopping him?" Clearly the answer to this question lay in an understanding of the forces that went beyond parenchyma and calories alone.

## Empathizing with the Patient's Anxieties about Meeting the Doctor

Typically, beginning students are so apprehensive about their own shortcomings and inexperience they, understandably, focus largely on themselves. Will they "blow" the interview? Will they miss getting that arterial puncture? Will the patient complain about them looking so young? Although such apprehensions are inevitable, it is often helpful for students to draw a conscious parallel: As apprehensive as the student may be, imagine how anxious the *patient* may be. The patient doubtless expects to see a young doctor, a concerned person, but one in a hurry, who will ask many questions. Will this young person approve of him? The last one got impatient when he could not recall the exact date his symptoms started, when he did not stick to the "important" details of his left lower quadrant pain. Will the student become physically disgusted by the smell from his infection? What will he think of the urine drainage bag dangling there below the sheets? If students can empathize with the enormous apprehensions a patient has about meeting a new doctor, some of their own self-consciousness may decrease. Furthermore, the appearance of anomalous reactions in such a setting can also be telling. As Engel pointed out in Chapter 3, patients who are not anxious, who immediately take the offensive, or who do not even seem to care are revealing important information about themselves.

## Developmental Stages

Erik Erikson[3] was one of the first to state what now seems obvious—that development and change do not cease at puberty. Rather, people undergo major developmental changes throughout their adult life. Since Erickson, important research has been done by Levinson[4] and Vaillant[5]. Much of this pioneering scientific work has also been incorporated into an excellent, timeless book by Gale Sheehy[6] titled *Passages*. It is extremely useful to familiarize oneself with this body of literature. Most students are young. Most of their patients are older. Although empathy, rapport, and understanding can bridge most gaps, students are helped immeasurably when they has some cognitive handles to help them understand what developmental issues a 40-year old, a 60-year old, or an 80-year old faces. Will the 50-year-old woman whom I am about to interview suffer from the "empty nest syndrome?" Will the high-level executive who is 48 and in the hospital for his first myocardial infarction be asking himself what he has really done with his life? People are almost always more complex than the paradigms we invoke to describe them. Nobody progresses predictably through locks in a canal. Nevertheless, there are normative stages that have now been well delineated, and, when applied flexibly, they can be very useful. Knowledge of them can be especially valuable to students who wish to form an empathic alliance with their patients—people so often different from students in background and age. Still, even during the early, often awkward moments when doctor and patient are trying to form a bridge, they have the most critical element of all in common: Despite differences in age, socioeconomic background, and life experience, both are human beings. Both know what it means to suffer; and whether either one admits it, both know, deep down, what it means to fear loneliness. Psychiatrist Harry Stack Sullivan once said, "We are all more human than anything else." This is true. A 25-year-old woman medical student raised in Massachusetts may be very surprised to discover how much she can understand about a 70-year-old Filipino immigrant dying of prostatic cancer—how much more than she might have imagined she possibly could. Our human capacity for empathy can be awesome and sometimes even a little frightening.

## The Patient Has a Life

Even the most isolated, down-and-out skid-row derelict has a life. He must have a place somewhere where he hangs out, and usually there are people he hangs out with; moreover, there are assuredly things that matter to him—maybe just a soiled snapshot or a tattered address book. Above all, everyone has memories and a past. Everyone had a mother and father—once. Everyone also has a future—hopes, aspirations, dreams, as well as illnesses and fears. Even our most anonymous patients have a life. Students should never forget that hospitals are very artificial environments. Hospitalized patients are stripped of their clothing, their wallets, and their jewelry. Favorite pipes and pictures are gone. We dress them in gowns and tell them to lie down flat. We isolate them from so much that makes each of them a person. Why we do this routinely to people is both curious and complex. In some ways, it seems necessary. Sometimes one wonders, though, if we perhaps do it also to protect ourselves emotionally. Maybe it is just too wrenching and frightening to see people so very sick in the full torrent of their humanness, and to think: They could be us. Whatever the reasons for our rituals, remember that the supine figure you see on a gurney under a sheet has a life, as surely as you or I. It is always worth inquiring into, for it is virtually impossible to treat someone inhumanely whom one understands, and sometimes our understanding itself can help immeasurably.

## FEELINGS

What do we do about feelings? In medicine, they are all over the place. Patients have them and we have them. Generally, we do not talk about them much. When they erupt, their occurrence often seems awkward, even guilt-laden: Witness the savage nursing station humor of house officers complaining on admitting night about getting another "hit." Similarly, patients may erupt suddenly into uncontrollable sobbing or rage. What do feelings have to do with medicine? Are they "scientific?" Engel addresses this question in Chapters 2 and 3 and concludes persuasively that understanding the feelings of doctor and patient is essential and amenable to scientific study.

Allow us to take the whole matter one step further. We propose that doctors who understand feelings—both their own and their patient's—are better doctors. They are better because they are able to comprehend what is truly important and therefore can provide more effective help. Empathy for our patients' feelings and insight into our own are not frivolous "window dressing," as some have made them out to be. We go even further: The failure of contemporary medical education to help students integrate their affect with their intellect may prove to be its greatest failing. Our profession is littered with casualties: doctors who are addicted, alcoholic, and divorced, or deeply depressed, disillusioned, and alone. For rare individuals, the apparent opportunity to deny all emotion may seem a welcome relief, but it is a dangerous denial—and one most of us do not welcome anyhow. For the vast majority of us, being in touch with our feelings and coming to peace with them is essential to our well-being. Patients who are not in touch with their feelings are thought to be more vulnerable to disease. We believe doctors, too, are at greater risk and for the same reason. We cannot continue to treat ourselves, much less our patients, like insensate machines. As educators, we have an absolute and urgent obligation to help physicians identify and cope with their feelings—in their patients and in themselves. We risk great peril if we do not achieve in this area.

### Feelings Are Useful

Feelings provide us with vital clinical data. To begin with, feelings are, biologically, very old, both phylogenetically and ontogenetically. They are the essential matrix for human bonding and socialization in our species, as essential to life as protoplasm. Phylogenetically and ontogenetically feelings originate first in lower mammalian forms and in infants. Ideas became attached to them later in evolution and development with the emergence of the neocortex. They are, in fact, essential. On a more day-to-day basis, each of us must come to grips with our own feelings if we hope to be effective as well as satisfied professionally. Above all, clinicians who are in good touch with their feelings possess a most wondrous and reliable diagnostic tool.

Let us return, at this point, to the case of the 430-pound man cited earlier. Recall that the students saw how many biopsychosocial influences were affecting this man, yet the situation remained very puzzling. Where were the feelings? He did not seem depressed, when he should have been. Where was the anxiety? After the interview, the students sat around a conference table yawning, cracking cynical jokes, and saying they wanted to knock off early that day. The preceptor began to write a list on the blackboard, a list of feelings the students were having. Among the feelings: hopelessness, despair, remoteness, and boredom. Above all, the feeling tone among the students was unmistakably dysphoric. Why?

It began to dawn on the students that they were having the feelings the *patient* should have been having. This discovery led to an interesting notion. The notion goes as follows: This man's entire family never recovered from the suicide of the 24-year-old son 4 years before. Instead of grieving or feeling depressed, the family's feelings seemingly went underground. In some complex way, the depression was hidden and then divided up among the whole extended family. The father ballooned into morbid obesity. The mother's voice became stifled. The students could only speculate about the family's many children, including the surviving children of the suicide; but, by the end of the discussion, a lot more was known. Using the data of their own feelings, the students were able to construct a decent, testable hypothesis to explain the bio-, psycho-, and social sequelae of this tragedy.

## Transference and Countertransference

Transference and countertransference, two rather lofty and formidable-sounding words, have suffered over the years from misuse and overuse. The terms originated in psychoanalytic theory, where they have specific definitions and applications. The concepts are nonetheless very useful, even if the argot has grown confusing. Rather than adding to the mess, consider a definition that is brief and intentionally quite simple: All human beings *transfer* things—feelings, attitudes, and expectations—they once had toward important people from their childhood, typically parents and siblings. Such transfers are probably ubiquitous, but often become highly prominent in the doctor–patient relationship, especially as it develops over time. Sometimes such transferences are problematic; often, they are not. Usually, however, it helps if they are understood. Some kinds of psychotherapy deliberately foster and then examine transferences as a major focus of treatment. This usually does not occur, however, in the typical doctor–patient relationship. Here is an extremely simple example of transference:

> A man of 36 grew up in a family where he felt his father was harsh and critical of everything he did. When this man, now an adult, began to develop signs of chronic obstructive pulmonary disease, his physician (a man his father's age) counseled him to stop smoking. When the patient did not do so, the physician admonished him about how really important this was for his health. The patient exploded angrily

and berated his surprised physician for nagging and belittling him, and not appreciating his efforts to stop.

This is *transference*. The patient acted as though the doctor was his father. In turn, the physician found *himself* reacting

*Countertransference*, strictly defined, is the reaction of a doctor to his patient's transference. In this case, the doctor had a reaction. He found himself disgruntled with his patient. He complained to a colleague about the patient's stubborn ingratitude, and especially the patient's unwillingness to let him be of help. This is countertransference; the doctor actually felt toward his patient like a disgruntled father. Many transference-countertransference reactions are far more complicated and subtle. Furthermore, it is quite possible for a physician to have *his own transference* to a patient. A physician's transference is considered countertransference among contemporary views. For example, if a young man is treating an older woman who reminds him of his caring mother, he may form a positive countertransference to *her*.

Students often quite properly protest the hazards of pseudopsychologizing. Sometimes students correctly assert feelings are straightforward and belong in the present. One student expressed the skepticism well: "Just because I was bored and grumpy today doesn't automatically prove that I'm having some kind of countertransference to my patient. Maybe I'm just in a bad mood. Maybe I was on call last night and didn't sleep. Maybe I had a fight with my wife."

Quite true! Yet it is still surprising how often these straightforward feelings can also originate in response to a person's *transference*. Of all his patients that day, for instance, why did the students get grumpy with *this* one? In any event, the most important skill involves being aware that transference often does occur. Patients are especially prone to developing strong transference feelings toward their doctors. Knowing that such feelings can and do happen, and having some notion that they might be transference, is more important than definition and jargon.

## Medical Slang

"Frequent flyers," "bounce backs," and "train wrecks." Let us be truthful. At some point, the most well-intentioned among us may conceivably use these denigrating terms or their equivalents, outrageous as that is. Thus, it is impossible to conclude a discussion of feelings in the doctor-patient relationship without talking about the frustrated, angry feelings medical students and house officers inevitably experience in the training hospitals where they spend so many crucial years. Typically this training occurs in large public hospitals, Veterans Affairs hospitals, jails, and city wards. Students are told they will have to take a lot of responsibility in these settings and see a lot of "pathology." Both statements are true. Frequently, however, students and young doctors are also assailed by a grim, raw, desperate, even hopeless side of human existence for which they were hardly prepared. Their sensibilities are shattered and overwhelmed by the seemingly endless procession of overcrowded wards, inadequate equipment, and haggard and overworked staff. Into these nightmarish environments flow severely ill people—people who are not just medically ill, but burnt out physically, crushed psychologically, defeated by life itself. In they pour like an interminable deluge—cases of hopeless alcoholism, drug addiction, brain damage, knife and gunshot wounds.

What one witnesses in these settings is *not* all of medicine or indeed all of life, but it is what young doctors may see day after day and night after night. Sometimes a benumbed feeling of nihilism sets in, even in the most sensitive of us. Very few of us can forebear endlessly or be so saintly that we never once call a patient by a disparaging label.

Still, we must ask why. As difficult as things may get, when we find ourselves using disparaging language toward our patients, we must ask why. Reflecting in this way provides insight that often helps. When we have a strong aversion toward a patient, usually something specific has gone wrong, beyond the general frustrations. Somehow, doctor and patient are failing to understand or empathize with each other at all. This is not always easy. Sometimes it may feel nearly impossible. Some patients *are* very far gone. Nevertheless, we have repeatedly seen instances in which a student or house officer expressed revulsion for a patient, not from nihilism, but because it seemed too painful to feel otherwise. The anguish seemed just too deep to bear and the reward for recognizing such feelings too miniscule, far too remote. Similarly, over and over we have witnessed patients suffering in these settings. More than a few are rude and hostile because underneath it all they are too terrified to hope, too frightened to reach out just one more time, to show their humanity, only to have it crushed again.

When you call someone a "train wreck" ask yourself why. It is almost impossible to loathe someone you understand.

## DENIAL OF DEATH

In Chapter 3, Engel observes that much of what we call "art," "intuition," and "bedside manner" are actually essential to the proper understanding of patients. He argues persuasively that, in this area, we probably have not been scientific enough. Yet, there is a widespread mythology that such matters are not amenable to scientific scrutiny. This mythology, coupled with our failure to effect such study, has had a disastrous effect on medical education. Engel believed this narrowness has evolved from the scientific model of Western medicine itself, which for centuries has been based on reductionism and the Cartesian mind–body dualism.

Yet could there still be another level to the problem? Why has modern medicine seemed so entrenched? At times, so stubborn? We personally suspect it has something to do with our inevitable proximity to what is most disturbing, mysterious, and impenetrable in life itself. Doctors are present when life is born. We are there when sane people go mad. We are there when death comes. By the nature of what we do, we are, inevitably and inexorably, tangled up with our patients in the crucible of life's most painful and agonizing questions. Above all, as mortal human beings ourselves, we doctors must nonetheless confront daily the most unimaginable yet undeniable truth of all: We all die. Without doubt, when we confront this reality in our patients, we are forced to make certain unavoidable inferences about ourselves. In Dr. B. J. Miller's TED talk on what really matters at the end of life,[7] he astutely identifies dying and suffering as the most apprehensive aspects of death—a necessary suffering that unites caregiver and care receiver whereby compassion is suffering together. *This is where healing happens.*

Centuries ago, before medicine was based on science, doctors were priests, shamans, and medicine men—witch doctors. Although they were endowed with the special respect due to those who have commerce with the ultimate mysteries of life and death, they were also lonely and set apart. In Keniston's words[8], they were members of a "feared and powerful guild."

Times have changed. Centuries have passed. Although some have wondered if a field can change so rapidly and constantly and still call itself a science, modern medicine is based indisputably on science and the scientific method. The dazzling technology that now surrounds us is not, in itself, dehumanizing. It is a monument to science and to the scientific method itself.

Yet for all of this, some things have not changed. People still die. Although we have advanced with astounding alacrity and success scientifically, we remain inevitably just as helpless, frightened, and befuddled as ever by mortality. For all our knowledge, we, too, remain deeply uncertain and alone.

We do not like this one bit, of course, and attempt with all our might to deny it. Probably the shamans and witch doctors did too. The causal connections our ancestors invoked had to do with angry gods and dangerous alignments of pathogeneses that originated in immune complexes, anaplasty, and genetic markers. We *are* much closer to the truth. We *are* being more scientific, but the ultimate riddle still eludes and torments us. The most unbearable truth has not changed. Maybe we doctors, if we are to become truly wise and at peace, must learn to accept that our intimate involvement with life's greatest mystery—death—commingles dramatically with the triumph of our advancing technology and expanding knowledge. We can do more and we know more, yet control of life's ultimate riddle remains beyond our grasp. We remain the descendants of shamans, and perhaps we should accept this and be proud.

Possibly, then, we can free ourselves and our students from the shackles of a narrow, dehumanizing view of people—a view that both denigrates science and ignores the existential curse and blessing of our calling. In the future, we will learn more and more about how people regenerate and degenerate, how they come into being and how they die. We will keep advancing on the truth—humane scientists, scientific human beings. However, we will all die, and our work has to do with this too. The renal failure in room 407 is you, me, all of us. If we are to achieve our ultimate stature as the noble professionals we can be, we must strive to study and learn always; but, we must realize that the very nature of our calling puts us in the eye of the hurricane. We deal with life's most inevitable, ineffaceable truth: our mortality. This is as true for us as it was for our noble shaman predecessors, who rubbed herbs in their hands, sang incantations, and searched for answers from dim and distant stars. We are closer, but still we search. By the very nature of science, there will always be this excruciating paradox. As doctors, the farther we push back the ocean of our ignorance, the more we will find ourselves still standing at the very edge of an unutterably beautiful and terrifying shore.

## REFERENCES

1. Reiser DE, Schroder AK. *Patient Interviewing: The Human Dimension*. Baltimore, MD: Williams & Wilkins; 1980.

2. Balint M. *The Doctor, the Patient, and the Illness.* New York: International Universities Press; 1964.
3. Erikson EH. *Childhood and Society.* 2nd ed. New York: Norton; 1963.
4. Levinson DS. *The Seasons of a Man's Life.* New York: Knopf; 1978.
5. Vaillant G. *Adaptation to Life.* Boston: Little, Brown; 1977.
6. Sheehy G. *Passages.* New York: Dutton; 1976.
7. Miller BJ. *What Really Matters at the End of Life?* TED Talk. Filmed March 2015. https://www.ted.com/talks/bj_miller_what_really_matters_at_the_end_of_life?language=en. Accessed August 14, 2016.
8. Keniston K. The medical student. *Yale J Biol Med.* 1967;39:356.

## SUGGESTED READINGS

Becker E. *The Denial of Death.* New York: Free Press; 1973.

Cassell EJ. *The Healer's Art: A New Approach to the Doctor–Patient Relationship.* New York: Penguin Books; 1979.

Quill T. Partnerships in patient care: a contractual approach. *Ann Intern Med.* 1983;98:228–234.

Rosen DH. Pursuit of one's own healing. *Am J Psychoanal.* 1977;37:37–41.

# 5

# THE PATIENT-CENTERED INTERVIEW

The purpose of this chapter is to describe an approach to talking with patients, one derived from principles inherent in the biopsychosocial model. What follows is not a lexicon of foolproof rules and techniques. In fact, the biopsychosocial model, by its nature, encourages a far more flexible approach to patients. It may be difficult to define precisely what constitutes a "biopsychosocial" interview, but a compendium of rote questions and rigid techniques it clearly is not. All too often, the latter is what students are accustomed to learning in its place. One should also realize that a chapter such as this is only an overview and cannot be fully comprehensive. Given these constraints, we delineate four key approaches to patient interviewing, approaches we view as fundamental to a full and effective understanding of all patients. Specifically, these four are the *science of observation, following the affect, the concept of process,* and the *A.R.T. of interviewing*. With some apprehension, we offer a section titled "'Strategies,' 'Hip-Pocket Standbys,' and 'Pearls.'" Although we are wary of oversimplifications, we see the need to provide at least some tricks of the trade. Finally, we offer a brief summation of what interviewing is and, just as important, what it is not.

## THE SCIENCE OF OBSERVATION

As Engel points out in Chapter 3, skills of observation can be greatly refined through education and practice. The fruits of such skills are valuable clinical data. They are essential in the medical evaluation and the clinical diagnosis. Some medical schools even have museum-based observational courses to help students hone their observational skills, with evidence to support improvement of medical students' visual diagnostic skills[1]—that of unbiased inspection and accurate reporting. Observational skills can be taught and can be learned.

Despite this logic, medical students are often astonished when an experienced interviewer draws conclusions from data that passed them by unnoticed. "How'd he figure that out?" Yet, 9 times out of 10, such students have actually managed to overlook evidence that lay conspicuously before them. The problem is not simply faulty memory. When students are reminded of a key observation that seemed to have eluded them, they typically respond with immediate recognition. They do turn out to have seen the critical incident. Somehow, though, they overlooked its significance—most likely because, lacking experience, they do not yet have a context into which the data fit, thus making them meaningful. As Engel points out, an experienced internist knows immediately what the sight of a patient sitting bolt upright in bed, struggling to breathe usually portends: congestive heart failure; the thought is almost a reflex. Less experienced students naturally lack such a matrix of repeated observation and experience, and therefore have more trouble anchoring the observable data to organizing concepts.

Still, everyone has to begin somewhere, and we urge students to heed this nostrum: Pay scrupulous, even compulsive attention to what happens first. The crucial significance of how interactions begin seems to be a highly replicable, indeed almost irresistible, human phenomenon. With astonishing predictability, patients reveal some of the most essential truths about themselves during the first minute or two of a new interaction with their doctor. Dr. Engel gives a beautiful example of this in Chapter 3. Recall the case of the retired businessman in a wheelchair who took over the seating arrangement and control of the microphone within the first few seconds of the interview. Engel remarks, "In this case, we first needed to establish whether this behavior constituted a specific reaction to the situation of being presented at rounds or if it reflected a more enduring personality style." Further inquiry supported the latter. As the patient described his hospital experience, the circumstances of his illness, his business career, his personal relations and family life, his satisfaction and frustrations, and his lifestyle, item after item emerged consistent with such a formulation (ie, the importance of control in this man's psychological functioning).

Like Dr. Engel, we should all be cautious of making too much out of too little. Students are especially leery of this danger and display appropriate skepticism toward those prone to "speculate." Still, with uncanny consistency, one finds that the behavior of patients during the early moments of an interview often does seem to predict and even summarize their general coping styles. This is in part because being interviewed is a challenge that demands coping. Therefore, make every effort to scrutinize all details of what transpires at the start. One cannot overestimate their value and importance. One clarification is required, however. Be aware that the interview does not actually begin with the doctor's formal invitation to start talking. Critical data, indeed often the *most* critical data, typically unfold before the interview has "officially" started. Keep your eyes peeled, beginning with the instant the patient comes into view.

Developing observational skills is actually not as formidable as one might think. Ultimately, all observable data must enter through one or more of the five senses. Physicians depend primarily on what they hear and see. Perhaps one also gets a "feeling" from time to time; and if such hunches are analyzed carefully, it becomes clear these "feelings" do not materialize from thin air. They are the product of a complex synthesis the doctor effects almost instantaneously from the data of the patient's expressions, sighs, body language, and other cues. It is true that increasing experience augments this ability to synthesize. Herein lie the rewards of sustained effort and clinical experience, but even beginners can learn much if they pay attention.

Take in everything. What happened during the crucial first minute? Was the patient sitting or lying? Did she lean forward or remain positioned as she was? What was the book that lay open on the man's lap? What did he do with it when he saw the interviewer first enter the room? How was the room decorated? What was the expression on the patient's face? How did it change? Were there any unusual odors? Does the patient have any get-well cards on his bedside table? Photographs of family? No? Why not? So much of importance is embedded in what people commonly pass off as trivial. If you were a novelist, you would invoke just such external details to symbolize the inner landscape of a character's mind. In reality, patients are not so different. They, too, reveal much in what seems to be commonplace. People classically reveal their more critical secrets in what is apparently trivial, habitual, and apt to go unnoticed. Look for these nuggets and you will find them. Above all, what *exactly* are the first bits of casual banter? These are always tip-offs.

One patient assented to be interviewed by remarking, "Sure! You can ask me anything you want except my bank balance!" Just a joke? It turns out not. Subsequent inquiry soon revealed that the most dramatic events in this patient's childhood had been his father's death when he was 6 years old. It occurred during the Great Depression and severe poverty followed. It turned out the patient was deeply chagrined because he had to be a patient in a public ward. In the past, he had been able to afford private care. Now, again, he was impoverished, just as he had been as a child. The tip-off was there—in the opening "joke."

After an initial period of vigilance, we then suggest a change in posture, one that may at first seem paradoxical. We explain its rationale when we describe the A.R.T. of interviewing. Let go. Adopt an even-hovering attention. Allow your thoughts and emotions (and those of your patient) to wander where they will. Trust in where such receptivity takes you. Students often ask, "How will I remember what happened?" In fact, if they pay careful attention to the interactions at the beginning, the rest can usually be recalled without difficulty.

## FOLLOWING THE AFFECT

Early in training, before a matrix of conceptual and clinical experience has been fully developed, the affect displayed by the patient is the student's most reliable organizer. Directing one's comments in relation to what the patient is feeling usually keeps patient and student on the right track, and also lends coherence to the student's own perception of the interview. Without attention to affect, an interview often seems fragmented, disjointed, and difficult to follow. Themes emerge, disappear, and reemerge. One minute the patient is talking about her liver; the next she is discussing a relative in Portland, Maine. The beginning interviewer, understandably, has trouble following these various threads. Almost always, however, an interviewer can perceive a distinct emotional tone that is fairly consistent throughout: depressed, anxious, reserved, seductive, and so forth. In addition, more rapid variations oscillate within the overall tone, similar to a brief series of musical notes played over the lingering resonance of a predominant chord. Both the chord and the notes are worth heeding. Also, the central emotional chord is usually sounded clearly and unequivocally during the first moments of the interview. Still, the notes that follow may range considerably. In a depressed patient, for example, one sometimes discerns shifts from anxiety to calm, from elation to despair, from hope to dejection.

Students' ability to keep track of their own feelings is equally crucial. Students also usually have a predominant emotional response to an interview—occasionally even the same thoughts and fantasies as their patients. Not long ago a group of students observed an interview with a dreadfully depressed, dying man. All 5 students quickly tuned out and indulged in essentially the same fantasy: getting out of the room. One daydreamed about dinner. Another thought about riding his bicycle. A third reminisced about a recent vacation. The content of the fantasies varied, but the theme was astonishingly consistent. Everyone felt restless and wanted to escape. By anchoring subsequent group discussion to these important data, we were able to develop a plausible hypothesis that explained the patient's severe isolation from his own feelings and experiences. The students had wanted to escape from the room because the patient had, in effect, already escaped—to some place very far away. Indeed, in his own mind, he was already gone—before the students had even gotten there! This dreadful truth was only accessible through an examination of the students' own feelings. This patient, in a sense, had already died.

Following the affect is also an effective way to keep an interview moving. Students who can stay with the patient emotionally by remarking from time to time, "That must have been sad," or "I bet *that* was frustrating," are usually able to help patients get to their most important concerns. Very often this intervention alone can bring insight and relief that are very therapeutic.

Students should also try to work up the nerve to *say* what the patient must be feeling, rather than asking patients what they feel when you think you know what they feel. It validates. Usually, students are empathically correct far more often than they give themselves credit for. Identifying an affect is almost always perceived by patients as supportive, not intrusive. Still, there seems to be a widespread myth to the contrary, that the "analytically proper" interviewer remains utterly neutral, open-ended, and completely unrevealing. Students must sometimes be helped to see past such clichés. Ponder the matter for a moment. If *your* mother had just died, which remark would *you* prefer: "You must be devastated" or "Tell me; how did her death affect you exactly?" Even if the student is wrong, the patient can always say no. When students are right, patients usually respond first with a yes, no, or maybe. It is in what follows this initial hedge that the students' correctness is actually affirmed or negated.

An inexplicable lack of affect on the patient's part is also important to keep track of. Why is a feeling *not* there when it should be? The same holds true for students as well. Why *does* the student feel bored when he "should" feel sad? This phenomenon is illustrated in Chapter 4 in the case of the 430-pound man.

Finally, although it may seem thoroughly obvious to experienced interviewers, students must be reassured that it is all right for them to *have* feelings! It is not easy for a beginning student to acknowledge boredom, disgruntlement, or dislike—much less sexual feelings, revulsion, or sadistic impulses. Usually, however, when students are reassured that such feelings are permissible (and come to appreciate that they may indeed disclose more about the patient than the student), the typical student quickly becomes able to identify and even delight in the broad range of emotions experienced during an interview. The key lies in assisting students to see that these emotions provide *valuable data about the patient*, not embarrassing revelations about the student.

## INTERVIEW PROCESS

The concept of *process* is essential to all good interviewing. This complex subject can be touched on only briefly here, and the explanation that follows must be regarded as introductory. There is a *process level to all* communication between people. It involves the rhythm, timing, and order in which themes, affects, ideas, and behavior arise during an interaction. An analogy to masonry is helpful. If the *content* of what the patient says forms the "bricks" of communication, then the process forms the mortar. Process is always present. In every interchange, people talk and listen; but as they do so, an endless series of silent questions, associations, and thoughts run through their mind, some at a more conscious level than others.

A useful analogy is to imagine you are at a cocktail party. For didactic purposes, imagine specifically that you are conversing with an interesting but unfamiliar stranger. You are curious, so you begin to make small talk. You talk about sports, current events, the weather. You ask each other about your interests. This is the surface of your interchange—the content. It is obvious, however, that something else is unfolding between the two of you below the surface. Behind the small talk, you are actively sizing each other up, revealing things about yourselves in some ways of which you are aware and, very possibly, in others of which you are not. What is going on between you at this level is *process*. You may be silently asking yourself: Is this person intelligent? Is he or she a good listener? What does he or she think of me? In such a social situation, you are not apt to pay too much attention to process, although it is there.

However, when doctor meets patient, the process level of communications between them becomes extremely important—a matter that goes far beyond a social interchange. So much of what is important to a patient is communicated in process, not content. A person who falls ill feels anxious, depressed, angry, irritable, hypersensitive, and frightened, among a host of other emotions that inevitably accompany significant illness. Often, however, the patient is not aware of these feelings, and just as often he is unable to express them to his doctor, at least not initially or straight out. The patient often has no choice but to communicate these vital concerns only at the process level. For instance, the following vignette illustrates a concern that is almost universal in patients: Can this doctor take care of me? Can I trust myself to be in her hands? Will she understand me? Sometimes patients are aware of these concerns, but more often not. Frequently they are just too afraid to admit them, even to themselves. Thus such thoughts almost never come up directly. They are communicated, instead, in process:

> A first-year psychiatry resident ushered his new patient down the hall to his freshly painted office for their first interview. The resident was clean but shaggy; he sported a full, reddish growth of beard and longish, although neatly trimmed, hair. He wore corduroy pants and looked, at best, 23. Money was tight at the time and, although he was impeccably clean, the back pockets of his Levi's were beginning to reveal holes. The soles of his boots had begun to wear through. They creaked with every step.
>
> The patient was 60; a meticulous man with silver-gray hair. He had paid scrupulous attention to all details of his dress. Even his shoes sparkled from a new shine. He had clearly gussied up for this occasion.
>
> As the patient followed his resident down the hall to the office, he remarked, "Hey, Doc! I think your back pockets are about to fall through. Your wallet's hanging halfway out!"
>
> The resident was initially tempted to go on the defensive, but he refrained. Once in the office, he waited for an opportune and tactful moment, and then remarked, "Bad

enough to get a resident, huh? Now a threadbare one to boot! Maybe you think I'm a green apple?"

"Nah," the patient replied initially, but soon he began to discuss his apprehensions. The resident was so *young*. The patient, on the other hand, was getting on in years. How *could* the resident truly understand his plight?

"I can see your point," the resident observed. "You're wondering if you've landed someone totally wet behind the ears. How could such a person understand the problems you face, especially those involved in a generation gap? I can see why you'd be feeling concerned."

"Well . . . yes and no." The patient finally responded. "The fact is, my wife and I have this problem . . . ."

The interview proceeded from that point quite smoothly.

The resident was no Svengali (manipulator). What he *did* do was to listen accurately to the interchange's process. Instead of reacting defensively to the content and its unmistakable accusation, he tuned in to the underlying concerns expressed in the process. He did so by heeding the following three questions:

1. Why is the patient telling me this *now*?
2. What is the patient telling me about his feelings *now*?
3. What is the patient telling me about his feelings regarding the relationship *between him and me now*?

A more extensive discussion of the interview process is beyond the scope of this text, but the concept is an important one. Understanding process takes practice, experience, and time. Still, students who do not master every nuance of the concept of process should not feel unduly discouraged. Usually, the mastery of precise observational skills, coupled with an awareness of affects (in both the patient and the student), enable most doctors and patients to communicate quite effectively. For students who wish to pursue the concept, a more detailed explanation is provided in Reiser and Schroder, *Patient Interviewing: The Human Dimension* (see Suggested Reading).

## THE A.R.T. OF INTERVIEWING

Consider for a moment the real implications of the biopsychosocial model, and something important becomes apparent: The importance of interviewing to patient care deserves its weight in interviewing texts and courses to capture the spirit and letter of the model to which we so bitterly pay lip service. Students should be open-minded to the bewildering array and variable quality of what is available. Some texts and courses offered narrow biomedical schemata, which provide often useful outlines for obtaining important details about signs and symptoms, but they leave out the person. Other texts and courses emphasize almost exclusively the psychosocial aspects of medicine, thus speaking eloquently of heartache but ignoring heart failure. All too often, students respond in suit, by dichotomizing instead of integrating. We have observed students respond to these courses and books, and their responses do indeed reveal a troubling bias. Students frequently end up regarding open-ended, psychologically oriented interviews as "my psychiatry course." Conversely, they refer to their biomedical training as "medicine." It is polarizing but understandable given the current circumstances.

A very pointed example of this transpired recently when we consulted with a junior medical student interested in family practice. He began by introducing his patient to us in the following manner: "Mr. Bartholomew," he began, "I hope you don't mind if we interview you for our psychiatry course." Thus, this student quite inadvertently betrayed the dichotomy in his thinking that Dr. Engel discussed earlier in Chapter 2 of this book. It is a false and highly destructive yet prevalent dichotomy: The "scientific" versus the "intuitive," "medical" versus "psychiatric."

Most medical schools in the United States have some kind of interviewing course. Typically, it is taught early, during the preclinical years, and it is not uncommon for it to be headed by a psychiatrist and mental health professionals. The intent of such courses is most surely noble. The idea originated in the reasonable wish to expose students to clinical contact with patients early on. Above all, such courses are meant to instill a humanistic appreciation for the patient as a person, not just as a vessel containing an interesting disease. Yet, our latest educational tactic may have backfired. All too often, students begin to associate humane, empathic attention to patients with "psychiatry." It is only a small step from this assumption to the conclusion that understanding the patient as a person has little to do with "real medicine," but is the province of "psychiatry"—just the opposite of what we educators intend. Furthermore, this very polarization is rife not only in the student's formal education but also in available textbooks.

We have observed the results of this polarization repeatedly in the apparent existence of an almost dual clinical personality among medical students. When medical students are on rounds with "psychiatric" types, they adopt, indeed find value in, the apparently more open-minded and holistic approach psychiatrists take to patients. Hours or even minutes later these same students go on rounds with their surgery or internal medicine team and revert with equal facility and conviction to a highly content-oriented, symptom-focused view of the same patient lying in the same bed. Why this occurs is addressed more fully in Chapter 2. What does it really mean? Suffice it to say that students are not acting as conniving double agents willing to go with one perspective at this instant, then attaching readily to another the next. Rather, it seems more likely that both approaches, in their commonly polarized forms, fail to help students integrate the benefits of each perspective into a unifying approach for interacting with patients. Platitudes aside, this integration is really not so simple. On the one hand, good doctors must be reflective, receptive, and sufficiently open and nondirective. They must allow the patient to open up. On the other hand, pressures of time and more important; the need for specific data pertinent to diagnosis requires that doctors "bird-dog" certain paths of inquiry with rigor and specificity if they hope to arrive at an accurate diagnosis. Both tasks, broadly construed, are essential to adequate and comprehensive management of any patient. Yet, effecting a bridge between interviewing process and content turns out to be one of the most difficult—although unquestionably one of the most important—skills a clinician has to master.

We cannot hope to redress this imbalance here. What we do hope to do in the following pages is to review briefly the conceptual bridge we find helpful in integrating these apparently disparate concepts: the A.R.T. of interviewing. The mnemonic device refers to three components of all good biopsychosocial interviewing: assessment, rankings, and transition. These terms are an attempt to offer a conceptual link between content and process during the clinical interview. Like all conceptual frameworks, this one should be viewed as a guideline and not as a set of rigid rules and nostrums. Really, there are no magical formulas in medicine, as much as we might wish them.

## Assessment

Because most doctor–patient interactions begin with a period of mutual assessment, how the doctor and patient size up each other is based on a host of factors, ranging from past experiences to the sense of intuition and "chemistry" that occur the moment these two critical partners in the dyad first meet.

The patient begins to assess the doctor from the moment he walks in the door. Is he young? Is he old? Does he look stern or kind? Is he clean-shaven and youthful or long-haired and bearded? Each of these clues filter through a matrix of past biases and experiences. For instance, a young patient who is a member of the counterculture is apt to react far differently to a long-haired resident than to a staunch-looking conservative, and so on. The factors that go into assessment are instantaneous, inevitable, and highly complex. To a large extent, these factors are initially nonverbal.

For doctors, assessment is more complex. They, too, have all the initial gut-level responses to their patients. In addition, they draw on the memory of many other patients they have seen before. From the beginning, doctors' assessments are based on clinical experience and personal memory. Is the patient cyanotic? Does she appear pale? Does he show visible pain? Is he moving all extremities? Finally, of course, astute clinicians keep in mind the kind of impressions they are making on their new patient. What does the subtlety in a patient's mannerism and expression reveal about how the patient is assessing the doctor?

Doctors are accustomed to a very focused and goal-directed approach to history taking. They try to go after the facts, to pursue a line of inquiry that yields the most data as quickly as possible. This is the reason why, traditionally, the chief complaint and identifying data come first, and why doctors then use these data as guidelines. At first glance, it hardly seems worthwhile to pursue an extensive history of joint distress in a patient whose chief complaint is chest pain. Still, the key to effective assessment is the clinician's ability to maintain a relaxed and open-minded receptiveness. After all, the chest pain might be the result of costochondritis or osteoarthritis of the spine. This is what Freud, long ago, called an "even-hovering attention." Such a stance is far less active than one to which clinicians are accustomed, and many doctors at all levels of experience find the restraint involved in this stance difficult. Yet, it is critical. Experienced clinicians are alert, yet quiet and receptive. Especially during the initial phases of the interview, they must be vigilant yet allow their mind to wander where it will. They may be struck by a smell or an unusual color in the patient's hair. They might find themselves curious about something they see at the patient's bedside. As the patient's story begins to unfold, many thoughts cross clinicians' mind. They associate to other patients and to diseases they have seen in the past, journal articles they recall, and syndromes they remember from grand rounds. Hypotheses begin to form, and their attention becomes progressively more active and directed. Obviously, this process depends on the extent of clinical and factual background the clinician possesses.

Beginning students cannot expect to "zero in" with the homing instincts of highly experienced clinicians. Yet, with increasing experience, hypotheses begin to enter students' mind during the assessment phase, and their attention begins to focus with increasing specificity and intensity. Obviously, this process of narrowing-in accurately improves with clinical experience, which brings to advanced clinicians a rich matrix of memories, cases, and factual knowledge. Regardless of one's level of experience, however, the diagnostic process should always begin with this phase of maximum open receptivity.

Perhaps it is partly beginning students' lack of clinical experience that leads them, early during training, to focus in too fast, resorting to lists and specific questions, and firing away aimlessly. Yet, even beginning students can learn the process of assessment. It is not a mysterious or an arcane art known only to the most advanced clinicians. Rather, it is a different way of being receptive to the empirical data of one's own observations—an approach that trusts the integrative abilities of the mind to sort through what is extraneous and to begin to discern the figure from the background of a clinical problem. Although experience and knowledge are crucial, even beginning students have a far richer matrix of memory and logic from which to work than they credit themselves with early in their training.

As we have suggested, assessment soon leads to an increased focusing-in as specific hypotheses are defined, refined, and zeroed in on rapidly. However, this is not truly a linear process in any simple sense. Even at a very advanced stage of the clinical interview, skilled physicians keep at least one part of their mind open. Even as they interrogate for pertinent specifics, another part of their mind hovers freely, still relaxed and ready to be taken by surprise. Assessment is a progression that occurs continuously throughout the diagnostic process with the patient, from beginning to end.

The highly nondirective stance of the assessment phase is also designed to assure patients of a sense of openness and trust. It encourages them to express any and all of their concerns, regardless of how trivial they might seem to them. For years, psychiatrists have known the importance of beginning an interview with open-ended, non-leading remarks. This is important in any interview, whether "psychiatric" or "medical"—terms we put in quotes because the biopsychosocial model views them as part of a continuum.

The extreme open-endedness of the initial assessment phase serves two purposes. First, it opens clinicians' mind to all data and possibilities. It permits the integrative and synthetic capacities of clinicians' own mind to begin to delineate critical features from a total gestalt. Second, it encourages patients to bring up whatever seems important. Sometimes this is an emotional concern; but, not infrequently, it reveals an important physiological symptom patients might have dismissed as too trivial to warrant mention. Often, these are the data that alert clinicians to where they should focus their attention.

Finally, although this hardly needs repeating, starting with an extremely open-ended question such as, "What sort of troubles have you been having?" or with merely a simple inviting gesture of the hand that tells the patient to commence, communicates the most important message of all: *You are my patient, but you are a person before you are a patient, and it is you, the total human being, who concerns me, not just your disease.*

## Ranking

As we suggested, ranking of hunches, hypotheses, and priorities occurs rapidly during the diagnostic interview. Although it is often not a conscious process in the minds of many clinicians, it goes on constantly. Ranking—zeroing in the lens from wide angle to a focused close-up—is a skill that increases with experience clinicians' assessments of a problem's medical urgency and, finally, clinicians' personal style. We feel that too many doctors tend automatically to rank biomedical problems at the top of every list. In doing so, they not only miss important biomedical data the patient may think "too trivial" or "unrelated" to bring up, but also they risk communicating to the patient that they are interested only in the physiology and organ systems affected by the disease.

There are, of course, medical emergencies in which a thorough medical history—at times even a true emergency triage—must be preempted by the immediate need for medical intervention. For instance, a patient with a possible myocardial infarction or one suspected of having a subarachnoid hemorrhage must be assessed rapidly from a biomedical perspective. A more holistic approach to the total person may have to wait, but not for long. Remember Mr. Glover's arterial puncture and cardiac arrest in Chapter 2.

Actually, such situations are far less common than is sometimes thought. Most patients do not present in a state of extreme medical or surgical emergency. Almost always there is time for an initial phase of open-ended assessment—a warm and inviting gesture of the hand that says, "Tell me your story. I'm interested. I will look you in the eye and care about whatever you bring up. It is *you* I wish to understand."

## Transition

Of the three skills contained in the mnemonic device, transitions are the easiest for even beginning students to effect. Smooth transitions are critical to a good interview and make the difference between a bewildering and even frightening experience for the patient, and one in which a sense of collaboration and trust begins to grow. Despite this, surprisingly few clinicians effect transitions with clarity, reassurance, and a clear sense of purpose the patient can grasp. Effecting transitions is really a matter of remembering to do it. We believe the reason clinicians often fail to do so is because they often forget how terrified and "in the dark" patients feel about their illness. For example, a clinician who suspects peptic ulcer disease but whose patient is currently talking about her fear of missing work may suddenly ask, "Have your stools ever turned black with this? Black, like tar?" The logic of such a question is obvious to the clinician, but the already frightened and bewildered patient may read far more ominous and confusing messages into such a radical shift. "The doctor is linking *my* problem, how can I manage to stay at work, with *black stools*. Does that mean I have *cancer*? Is it a sign that I may not live?" Obviously, these apprehensions are always present. This is the reason why good clinicians must always pay attention to all of their patients, not just to a part of them. Smooth transitions can help. For instance, the doctor cited in this hypothetical example could have changed the subject by saying, "I'm sure you are concerned about getting back to work without jeopardizing the project you're working on. Let's get back to that; but, I would like to turn my attention now more specifically to this pain you've been having in your abdomen, where you pointed a few moments ago. Let me ask you some specific questions that may help me understand the nature of the problem. Have you ever noticed any change in the color of your stools?"

The real trick to effecting transitions is to remember that a patient is not a physician and cannot read your mind. Therefore, when you shift lenses, whether it be to zoom in or pan out, share these transitions with the patient: Explain why you are shifting your line of inquiry at that particular point. It sounds simple, and it is, yet it is frequently overlooked at the expense of needless patient suffering.

## Comments on A.R.T.

We have invoked the A.R.T. mnemonic device to delineate the three phases that we believe occur in all doctor–patient interactions. We feel there is considerable conceptual advantage in discussing them separately. Students should remember, however, that these three phases do not proceed in any simple lock-step fashion, with one phase leading neatly to the extent. Actually, all three processes go on constantly and indeed simultaneously.

The A.R.T. paradigm was developed to help interviewers establish an alliance with their patients that permit them to obtain important data in all three sectors of the biopsychosocial sphere. Its usefulness naturally increases with growing clinical knowledge and sophistication, but we believe the framework may be useful from the onset of clinical learning. Above all, the goal of this and kindred paradigms should be viewed as heuristic rather than prescriptive. Beginning students, especially, should not expect of themselves a matrix of clinical experience that is not yet there. Beyond this, translating the biopsychosocial model into a readily applicable method of ongoing patient care has not yet been fully achieved. There is some promise with an evidenced-based, patient-centered method using this model summarized in a commentary piece by Smith[2] et al. (authors of the method), but the field awaits further synthesis.

## "STRATEGIES," "HIP-POCKET STANDBYS," AND "PEARLS"

Every patient is different, and every doctor–patient relationship is unique. Most students appreciate this, but they also want answers: pearls, mnemonics, and tricks of the trade. Clinically, all students get into jams, and they want to know methods for getting out of them. Understanding is great, students say, but they also want some specific plans of attack and ways to get out of a pickle. Fair enough. But students must also remember there are no foolproof tricks. From their own experience, they know full well that the very worst doctors are the ones who have memorized a dozen "tricks" and proceed to apply them with procrustean monotony to every patient. Still, there are some tricks of the trade; and with these cautionary observations, we offer some "pearls." Remember, though, they are not foolproof, nor are they ever a substitute for understanding.

1. *Dress professionally.* Uyen's mother asked in Vietnamese, "Do you not respect your patients [given her no makeup, no-frills appearance on a day she was running late]?" It gave Uyen pause. She was in professional attire as expected by her workplace's dress code, but one detail did not go unnoticed. She initially wrote it off as a very conservative perspective by her mother, but the comment lingered. Perhaps not all patients would perceive this as a lack of respect, but we should aim to eliminate as many barriers as possible to establishing rapport. Beyond paying attention to how we present ourselves with respect to physical appearance (grooming, hygiene, attire), we should pay equal attention to our posture, mannerisms, and tone of voice, as well as body language (more on this later). For medical students, it is a courtesy to your patient for you to don your white coat, and it identifies you as being associated with the healthcare team. It also reduces the disadvantage your relative youth may impose. Patients feel reassured, not deceived by the white coat.
2. *Respect confidentiality.* The Health Insurance Portability and Accountability Act of 1996 guides us to safeguard patient's medical information, but you will see occasions when your professors and peers do not. We caution you not to succumb to the pressures of others who are in breach of confidentiality. We have a legal obligation as well as an ethical one. Confidentiality is stressed in the Hippocratic oath, in addition to *do no harm*. Our patients are too vulnerable to be harmed in any way.
3. *Be yourself.* Authenticity matters. Patients are astute in knowing when you are trying to be someone other than yourself. Do not inhibit yourself by trying to imitate some caricature of a pseudo-Freudian statue. Humor is great medicine when appropriate (and a healthy, mature defense). If patients joke, and it's funny, it's okay to laugh! Sharing a detail or two about your personal life may help build rapport and engage patients. Use your judgment. There are also times when it is appropriate, even indicated, to touch patients or hold their hand. If you are naturally reserved, do not be phony, but do not be afraid to reach out and be human either. Remember, however, that physical contact is a very potent "drug" with side effects. It takes experience to know when to touch and when not to. However, you will never learn if you always keep your hands in your pockets. Remember also, though, that an understanding expression and kind word, spoken softly and with empathy, can also "touch" a patient—sometimes far more deeply than any pat on the back. Always guide yourself by asking: Am I doing this for me or for my patient?
4. *Be warm but not contrived.* Express your warmth in a way that sincerely reflects your own personality. Do not develop a repartee of glib social patter. Small talk about weather, sports news, or current affairs may be an opening, but is no substitute for real warmth and interest in your patients. They have entrusted themselves to your care. The matters they face are serious.
5. *Let patients cry.* Crying is a powerful release and can be healing, especially if your empathy has helped them to feel understood. If you were this patient, you might cry, too—alone in the hospital, sick, confused, in tremendous pain. Patients' tears often represent the highest tribute they can pay you. They would not cry in your

presence if they did not feel understood and safe. Give them some space without interruption. The same general principle applies to other strong affects—rage, fear, love. In general, if feelings are being expressed at a reasonable decibel level, let your patients emote.

6. *Think of your patient in developmental terms.* Read Levinson[3]'s book *The Seasons of a Man's Life* or Sheehy[4]'s *Passages*. It is difficult to know at 25 what it must be like to be 60. It helps to learn, and there are some good books to help you out.

7. *Remember that the patient is more scared than you are.* Patients may be nervous about meeting you, and—remarkable as this may seem—they may be even more self-conscious than you are. They *need* you. Never forget for a minute how important it is for patients to want to make a good impression on you. Do not let your own self-consciousness blind you to your patients'.

8. *Pay attention to feelings.* Pay attention to your patients' and *your* feelings. They are the best compass you have. You will get better at this as you mature clinically, but, at worst, you will probably turn out to be better at it than you think. Rest assured, patients tell you if you are wrong.

9. *Tell a patient what you think he is feeling.* Do not play 20 Questions. This is one of the most common errors made by beginning clinicians, including beginning psychiatrists. Think of yourself for a moment. Imagine you are in the hospital for an exploratory laparotomy. You might have cancer. Who would be more helpful for you? A physician who says to you, with an expression of concern, "This must be frightening for you" or a physician who rubs his perfectly manicured beard and, with an expressionless face, asks, "How do you feel about your upcoming operation?" Over the years, fewer scenes have been more painful to us than the spectacle of a young psychiatrist asking a visibly suffering patient, "How do you feel?" This "neutrality" is a myth that somehow has gained widespread and undeserved credulity.

10. *Share your joys, and your pain, with a friend.* Please reach out to your husband, wife, lover, friend, support group. If you need a psychotherapist or meditation teacher, see one. Do not be a "lone soldier." Medicine is an incredibly intense undertaking, which can engulf you if left to your own devices. Approximately 300 to 400 physicians die by suicide each year in the United States.[5] Doctors who end up killing themselves are usually the ones who tried to endure the pain alone. It just is not necessary. Do not let deluded "stalwarts" convince you otherwise.

11. *With patients, who you are is far more important than the act you put on.* "Patients do not care how much you know until they know how much you care,"—a statement often attributed to Theodore Roosevelt. This applies at all levels of training. As a medical student, show some self-compassion if you bumble your way through an interview or a procedure, because your patients will likely understand if they know you care. Certainly, be prepared in your studies and practice to minimize subjecting your patients to unneeded emotional or physical pain. If a resident or intern tries to make you do something you cannot, then ask for help. Most patients will trust and respect you, even if you stumble over your questions and shine the ophthalmoscope in your own eyes—if they sense you care. It is true that more experienced clinicians can often instill greater confidence in their patients. Medicine

is a field in which one does get progressively better. Still, most of your patients will know what really matters and will let you be their doctor even if you do stumble on your own shoelaces a time or two.

12. *When an interview bogs down, try repeating the patient's last words.* Psychologist Carl Rogers[6] first introduced the technique of repeating the last few words a patient says to encourage the patient to open up. Some interviewers try to get away with doing nothing *but* this, which then loses its usefulness. However, repeating the patient's words *can* be remarkably effective. It is as close as you will come in interviewing to a sure-fire trick. However, be mindful not to overuse. An alternative silence can also accomplish the same (see no. 14).

13. *Ask the "unaskable."* If you are in touch with your own feelings and those of your patients, you may realize when they are very scared or depressed. It may even occur to you that they consider life is not worth living and have thoughts of ending it. Tragically, some patients do. Most do not, but the real tragedy is aloneness; many think about death but feel they cannot tell anybody. It is a devastating, guilty loneliness. It is your duty to ask, with tact and sensitivity—not as part of a checklist as you review systems. Similarly, if you suspect child or elderly abuse, alcohol misuse, illicit drug use, or sexual concerns, it is your duty to ask the unaskable. If approaching such sensitive topics is not taught formally in didactics, then it is incumbent upon you to ask your intern, resident, and/or attending. Ask how they would make such inquiries, or—better yet—observe and take note of their interviewing skills and incorporate them into a script that suits you. Patients usually open up with relief, even gratitude, and often let you know if you should back off.

14. *Learn to be quiet.* When patients come to a point in their discussion with you where they are getting to uncomfortable material, often they fall silent. Silence is socially awkward, but as a professional, you can learn to use it. When patients fall silent, go ahead and be silent too! Yes, the pressure *does build*. It feels awkward. Seconds feel like hours. Soon enough, however, your patient will continue speaking, and usually they go on to tell you what really hurts. People make fun of psychiatrists for their legendary silences. Sometimes psychiatrists do overdo it, but in general they are on to something. The taboos of normal social discourse affect us all, and we all share the impulse to avoid silence. Observe, for example, the rapidity with which someone always jumps in at a dinner party with idle chitchat or other banter the moment a group falls silent. The doctor–patient relationship is no Sunday brunch. It is true that repeated, sadistically protracted silences reflect serious insensitivity, but most doctors would do well to listen more and talk less.

15. *Pay attention to body language.* Body language is one of many avenues patients use to communicate. This subject has received considerable attention in both medical and lay publications, with training courses available to help one interpret body language to improve nonverbal communication. It is a very important way in which patients (and doctors) express themselves. Unlike the tongue, the body seldom lies. Research has even suggested that body cues provide more valid data than facial cues alone in identifying emotions accurately.[7]

Body language at the beginning of an interview is particularly revealing. Observe how patients position themselves and move at the outset of the interview.

Watch the way they sit or stand, the way they seek or avoid direct eye contact. Despite the proliferation of books on the topic, most students know innately what one posture is "saying" in contrast to another. Phylogenetically, body language is an old and highly reliable form of communication. We still use it. The trick, as with other observational skills, lies in being *conscious* of what we observe and in allowing ourselves to *think* about it.

As students advance, especially if they learn how to listen to the process of communication as well as the content, body language becomes simply one of the many avenues through which patients communicate their concerns. However, it remains a perfectly reliable and legitimate source of understanding. It is a language that is always present and, by its nature, one incapable of dissembling.

16. *Start broadly and focus gradually.* At the outset, it is rarely necessary or wise, to focus narrowly on any predetermined agenda. Allow patients a few minutes to bring up whatever is on their mind. Listen. There is ample time to focus on specifics as the interview proceeds. This concept is amplified in the previous discussion of A.R.T. The only possible exception to this principle is a medical emergency, during which a rapid, focused assessment of worsening physical symptoms is imperative.

17. *The patient-centered approach is always right.* Much has been written about so-called "difficult" patients. Typologies have been developed to differentiate these types of clients and strategies have been developed for managing them. These categories can be very helpful, although people are always more complicated than our most elegant schemata. Actually, there is one thing these very different and difficult patients share. One way or another, they all faze interviewers and, in some way, knock them off balance. How this manifests can vary greatly—an impossible request, a refusal to cooperate, seductiveness, monotonous complaining. Regardless of the presentation, the effect is always to disarm and put interviewers on the defensive, which can lead to some terrific impasses and occasionally to no-win situations between doctor and patient. Interviewers in these situations often feel trapped by two impossible choices, neither of which will work. On the one hand, they can get defensive, which simply inflames these patients. On the other, they can try to be conciliatory and give in to the demand, but this invariably leads to repeated demands in an escalated way. A better approach, odd as it may seem at first, is to agree with these patients. Let us look at a simple example to illustrate this point:

Mr. Penderhughes is a hostile 50-year-old senior department store manager who never seems to stop complaining about something being wrong with the way the hospital is treating him. When the student approaches him to request an interview, Mr. Penderhughes barks, "You're another one of those medical students, aren't you? I'll be damned if I'm going to be a guinea pig in this hospital!"

Clearly, arguing back is not going to work. There's the reasonable approach of simply apologizing (even if not at fault) to mitigate the situation. For Mr. Penderhughes, obsequious apologizing will not work because he will stonewall the student. Of course, the student—in some settings at least—can back off and forget the whole mess. Let the intern take care of it. However, the time comes, soon enough, when the student *is* in charge. A better approach with Mr. Penderhughes is to *agree*.

"You're right, Mr. Penderhughes," the student might respond. "You have been an asset to help us learn from the time you were admitted, but I can see how you view it as being a guinea pig."

Some people call this technique "going with the resistance," or "paradoxical intention." It's in the spirit of patient-centered care and in a similar vein to "the patient is always right." We may not always understand these patients' complaints or their reasons for them, but surely they *have* them, so it may be better to agree and take the stance of humility.

This technique is by no means foolproof, but in a surprising number of instances, these patients begin to talk. Mr. Penderhughes may begin, albeit angrily, to tell the student about all the people who promised him help, only to fail him in the end. A depressed woman with Crohn's disease may sigh wearily and begin to speak of the numerous doctors and treatments that have already failed because her disease is "hopeless anyway." Such talk may not be pleasant stuff, but at least the doctor–patient interaction has begun. This approach works far more often than one might imagine.

18. *Manage expectations with time.* Start the interview by telling patients how much time is allotted for the appointment (because time varies from new to follow-up appointments). Apologize in advance in the event you have to interrupt to streamline the interview. This helps you pace yourself as well as helps patients prioritize any concerns early on to avoid "door knob" questions.

19. *Provide a summary and make time for questions.* Endeavor to summarize patients' presenting problems and their clinical impact, and validate any feelings elicited. This goes a long way in patients feeling understood and heard, and segues nicely into discussions of preliminary diagnoses, prognosis, and plan of care. At the end of the interview, ask your patients whether they have any questions or concerns. If you suspect they may not have followed the entire plan of care outlined, ask them to repeat it back to you or, better yet, write the plan down for them.

20. *Mistakes are inevitable, so consider how to learn from them and perhaps offer a sincere apology.* Doctors are not immune to being human. Medical errors will occur and may lead to an unfavorable outcome. Morbidity and mortality conferences exist in surgery and other specialties, but the culture in which we practice does not readily provide a space to acknowledge and learn from mistakes. Nevertheless, speak about them openly in a manner to be supported. Every medical student should watch emergency physician Dr. Brian Goldman's TED talk[8], in which he speaks candidly on this topic and what it means to be a redefined physician—that of acknowledging the limits of being human, that of acceptance when mistakes are made, and that of learning from what occurred to teach one another.

When mistakes happen, consider a sincere apology. This can go a long way to preserve the therapeutic relationship. Although existing research suggests apologies in the context of medical errors can benefit both patients and providers, in practice it is done infrequently.[9] The fear of potential litigation is cited most commonly as a barrier, although the link is not clearly established. This is a complex issue given the litigious landscape in which we practice. Therefore, seek input from your attending and risk management team.

## THE HEALING PROCESS

At heart, it seems to us that the doctor–patient relationship is always precisely that—a *relationship*, a mutual process, a sharing that is both intimate and complex. We so seldom speak of mutuality, so rarely acknowledge that we and our patients are actually in the same boat. Let us face the truth: We are, in fact, constantly collaborating with our patients, whether to obtain a history, treat an illness, or find the courage to face life's most cruel and puzzling mysteries. Yet, so often, we talk and act as though doctors were somehow exempt from the very laws of nature—spared the vicissitudes of life and death. We pretend, instead, to be distant gods. We like to hover, curious and inquisitive but detached, over the Petri dish of life, occasionally adding a drop from the end of our very long emotional pipettes. Why do we pretend we are so different from our patients? Is it possible that, at times, we deny our humanness because our work exposes us to a side of humanness that can frighten us desperately? We think so. This is all terribly hard to admit, and to admit so relentlessly, so endlessly, so daily. We, too, get sick, get angry, grow old. We die. Perhaps this sounds morose, but we personally view the matter very differently. We believe doctors can find the greatest meaning and joy in life when they admit that they, too, are a part of the most fascinating, terrifying, and unexplored continent of all—the human continent.

Hopefully, we will become ever more discerning in the study of our own humanness. Hopefully, the power and the beauty of our calling will come from the humility and compassion we bring to this quest.

## REFERENCES

1. Naghshineh SL, Hafler JP, Miller AR, et al. Formal art observation training improves medical student' visual diagnostic skills. *J Gen Intern Med*. 2008;23(7):991–997.
2. Smith RC, Fortin AH, Dwamena F, Frankel RM. An evidence-based patient-centered method makes the biopsychosocial model scientific. *Patient Educ Counsel*. 2013;91:265–270.
3. Levinson DJ. *The Seasons of a Man's Life*. New York: Knopf; 1978.
4. Sheehy, G. *Passages*. New York: Dutton; 1976.
5. American Foundation for Suicide Prevention staff. *Physician and Medical Student Depression and Suicide Prevention*. American Foundation for Suicide Prevention. https://afsp.org/our-work/education/physician-medical-student-depression-suicide-prevention. Accessed August 14, 2016.
6. Rogers C. *Client-Centered Therapy: its current practice, implications, and theory*. Boston: Houghton Mifflin; 1951.
7. Hillel A, Yaacov T. Body cues, not facial expressions, discriminate between intense positive and negative emotions. *Science*. 2012;338 (6111):1225–59.

8. Goldman B. *Doctors Make Mistakes: Can We Talk about That?* TED Talk. September 2011. https://www.ted.com/talks/brian_goldman_doctors_make_mistakes_can_we_talk_about_that. Accessed August 14, 2016.
9. Robbennolt JK. Apologies and medical error. *Clin Orthop Rel Res.* 2009;467(2):376–382.

## SUGGESTED READINGS

Binger C. Why the professor fell out of bed. *Harpers.* 1947;195:337–342.

Morgan, WL, Engel GL. *The Clinical Approach to the Patient.* Philadelphia: W. B. Saunders; 1969.

Reiser DE, Schroder AK. *Patient Interviewing: The Human Dimension.* Baltimore, MD: Williams & Wilkins; 1980.

Rosen DH. Modern medicine and the nature of the healing relationship. *Humane Med J Art Sci Med.* 1989;5:18–23.

Snow CP. *The Two Cultures and the Scientific Revolution.* New York: Cambridge University Press; 1961.

Szasz TS, Hollender MH. A contribution to the philosophy of medicine: the basic models of the doctor–patient relationship. In: Millon T, ed. *Medical Behavioral Science.* Saunders, Philadelphia: Saunders; 1975:585–92.

# 6

# THE EXPERIENCE OF ILLNESS AND HOSPITALIZATION

To become ill, even slightly so, is always disruptive. We forget just how disruptive, of course, as soon as we recover; but think back and recall how troublesome your last cold actually was. A cold is trivial enough, yet at the infection's height you probably could not think clearly and felt too uncomfortable to enjoy reading, music, friendship, or even food—and this was just a cold. When a person enters the realm of more serious illness, wrenching disruptions and profound feelings of anxiety and loss are inevitable. Moreover, illness forces change in a person: altered expectations, dashed hopes, and a fragmented self-image. Ill people do not choose to change; they must. Yet, just as the Chinese symbol for crisis represents both danger and opportunity, illness can be an important, although unwelcome opportunity for new strength and inner growth, as well as a terrible threat. In this chapter, we cover in a broad overview some of the key concepts involved in understanding how patients experience illness and hospitalization, including the stages of illness, the experience of illness depending on who the person is, the challenges of illness, coping mechanisms, and so-called "problem patients."

## STAGES OF ILLNESS

Much attention has been given to the phenomenon of health-seeking behavior. What are the factors that lead people to identify themselves as patients? What motivates them to call a doctor for an appointment or to drive to an emergency room and seek medical care actively? Obviously, the answer is multifaceted and based on much more than the mere presence or absence of a given symptom. *Who* these people are is critical, as is their previous experiences with illness, their perception of doctors, the reactions and pressures of their family, and the symbolism of the symptom; these and many other influences go into any person's decision to seek help. To give just one example: An otherwise healthy adolescent might well be apt to ignore increasing thirst and a pressure to urinate unless he knows from what had happened previously to his sister how diabetes can first present. Conversely, few people would ignore the appearance of blood in their urine. The cause of blood in the urine might not be as ominous as the appearance of thirst and urinary frequency. Yet, here the symbolism of the symptom becomes very potent. Few people could see blood in their urine without becoming alarmed. In most cases, this alarm would drive them to seek medical attention, even if the ultimate cause of the hematuria turned out to be less serious than the discovery of juvenile-onset diabetes.

Health-seeking behavior is also affected greatly by the emotional, psychological, and social context in which physical symptoms appear. As we have emphasized so many times in this book, a complete and thorough physician *must* include an assessment of these as part of the evaluation of any patient. Consider, for example, the hypothetical case of two young mothers. Both are 26 years old and both have 5-month-old nursing infants. Let us assume also that both have "identical" headaches located in the same place, with attributes that are completely alike. Yet, the headaches turn out to be vastly different for each when we consider the life setting in which they occur. Mother A feels overwhelmed currently and terrified. At times she feels suicidal. This is something she has not told anyone and does not tell her doctor voluntarily unless she discerns how distraught she is and tactfully, but firmly, inquires into her depression. This mother will tell her physician (*if* she asked) how, everyday, she struggles with an urge to beat her screaming, colicky infant. On several occasions, in fact, she has come close. She is terrified that the urge will get out of hand. Nor would such an occurrence be foreign for her. As a young child she was beaten repeatedly and severely by her own mother. When she calls her physician for an appointment, however, she reports only "headaches."

Mother B, our other woman with headaches, can fortunately be dealt with more briefly. Her life is reasonably happy, her family setting is safe and secure, and she is well integrated psychologically, with a stable sense of self-esteem. She does not, in fact, think to call the doctor. Two aspirin tablets seem to do the trick and she never actually picks up the phone.

Identical headaches, but vastly different problems. To discern this, however, physicians must appreciate their patients' difficulty at different levels of the systems hierarchy. A note in the chart that reads "tension headaches likely, rule out CNS tumor or migraine" is just not adequate. Yet, some physicians limit the focus of their inquiry to just this degree. If a doctor were to put on such blinders in her assessment of Mother A, she would doubtless leave the office with a muttered, "Thank you, doctor," most likely with a prescription in her hand (that may never be filled, much less taken or, conversely, might be filled and taken all at once). She will have left with her real pain unexpressed, possibly to go home and explode. And the doctor might well believe that she has a satisfied patient and has done a competent job.

Finally, we wish to emphasize one subtle, yet critical point regarding the management of these "identical" headaches. The proper intervention is derived from an understanding of systems theory; it is not a matter of "bedside manner" or "clinical intuition." Nonsystems-oriented physicians might or might not see value in inquiring about patients' circumstances and life. They might think of this as interpersonal warmth, humanism, viewing the patient holistically—or they might consider such matters basically trivial. Physicians who understand systems theory know differently; viewed from this perspective, understanding patients comprehensively is essential. A systems approach makes it clear that mother A's headache is affected, possibly even precipitated, by the emotional stresses she faces. To inquire of her about these is not being "kind" or "sensitive," it is being diagnostically complete— To reiterate: changes at any one level of the systems hierarchy invariably affect the functioning of systems at many other levels of the hierarchy. The rage, frustration, and despair that mother A feels at the level of the two-person system (she and the child) and at the family level of the system (Where is her husband? What roles has her own child abuse played in her life?) have effects at the organ system level. The precise nature of these effects has yet to be well delineated, although research continues to be promising. For example, high levels of stresses (and chronic stress) such as the ones mother A is experiencing are reported in patients with migraines, and is said to alter protective adaptive responses of the brain with resultant pathophysiological changes in brain structure and function, including immunological changes.[1]

The reason why it is so critical to grasp the highly interactive nature of different levels in the systems hierarchy is because, without such an understanding, physicians are not able to prescribe the best treatment for their patients. For mother A, this treatment obviously involves more than the prescription of pain tablets. It is true that Valium may relieve her muscle spasm and codeine, the subjective experience of pain, but these interventions do nothing to alter the disturbances at higher levels in the systems hierarchy that are precipitating the problem. The physician must help mother A to deal with her concerns about her parenting capacities and the current relationship with her husband and child, whether through referral to a psychotherapist for individual therapy or through family and parenting support services in the community. It is the only rational treatment strategy to be applied in this case. Finally, physicians who truly understand systems theory (after proper diagnosis and treatment at all levels of the system) do understand *why* the headache got better—and why the 20-minute counseling session the therapist conducted with mother A and her husband was a potent therapeutic intervention resulting in effective treatment of her headaches and painful situation.

Given the contextual nature of illness and the importance of viewing it from a systems perspective, it should be possible to conceptualize an evolving illness broadly, encompassing more than pathophysiology alone. Reiser and Schroder[2] proposed that one way to conceptualize reactions to illness is to view serious illness as a *development crisis*, occurring within the overall context of a person's life. From such a perspective, illness may be viewed as a new, and sometimes critical, challenge to a person's homeostasis and sense of identity. As this crisis evolves, three important states in that evolution may commonly be discerned: *awareness, disorganization, and reorganization*. In the discussion that follows, we delineate some important characteristics of each of these stages. Bear in mind, however, that people are inevitably more complicated than the schemata we use to categorize them. Still, there may be some value in recognizing that illness is an evolving process with often critical implications for human development, and not just some unfortunate moment frozen in time, quickly to be forgotten.

## AWARENESS

Awareness, above all, is characterized by *ambivalence*. As it begins to dawn on a person that something is wrong, whether it to be in the body or mind, a terrible conflict sets in: Does one struggle to deny the problem and pretend that nothing has changed? Or does one acknowledge the dreaded truth and begin to seek answers? Reason and logic notwithstanding, most people seem to do both, either simultaneously or in rapid succession. One moment typical patients dismiss the problem altogether: "It's just a cold."

The next they are convinced of the worst: "I know it's cancer." This is a period of great anxiety and bewilderment. Often it is mercifully brief. The symptoms abate, normal functioning returns, and people "forget" that anything ever was, or could be, seriously wrong. Fortunately, it did turn out to be just a cold! Some illnesses, however, are more serious and do not go away. People so beset, so frightened and conflicted, soon become our patients—a role transition that is far from painless or simple.

Why not use the more simple and more common term *denial* in place of the concept of *awareness* and *ambivalence* about knowing the truth? After all, we commonly hear that people early in an illness use "denial"—and indeed, they do! The problem with the term is its static, nondynamic connotation. When people use denial, they never do so completely or with total success. This is because denial is only *half* the patient's conflict. People *wish* to know the truth, even as they fight to *deny* the truth. The concept of denial is, ultimately, too simplistic to describe what patients experience at this stage of illness. During the stage of awareness, one part of the person *needs* to know, *craves* to know, and *prays* to know. Simultaneously, another part of the person needs *not* to know, craves *not* to know, and prays *not* to know. Both parts are equally intense and, during the stage of awareness, are in active conflict with each other.

Most of you can appreciate what the stage of awareness is like for a seriously ill person by recalling the fleeting health worries we all have had at one time or another when some "trivial" symptom has appeared. Medical students reading this book especially should have no trouble understanding this state. For a period during their education, every new disease students learn about tends to induce in them the very understandable fear that they might now get it. Although this is sometimes laughingly called the medical student's "hypochondriasis," it is actually a painful and frequently inevitable part of learning to be a physician. Students so beset can understand patients' ambivalence. "That bump on the elbow *probably* is just a bump"; but still, the thought intrudes, "It could be *cancer*." "That nosebleed I got doesn't mean I have leukemia. After all, I've gotten nosebleeds like this since I was a kid." Yet, then, the more dreaded thought: "Leukemia!" To empathize fully with patients' experiences, students must only imagine that the bump does not go away but grows bigger, that the nosebleeds become more intense and frequent. Now, denial begins to fail. Something is amiss! Something is very wrong. The intense anxiety and marked ambivalence patients experience during this stage clearly can become quite excruciating. Finally, sometimes the struggle to continue to deny can have tragic consequences, as in patients who deny symptoms of a myocardial infarction and fail to get to the hospital on time or patients who fail to get a mass sampled before it metastasizes and spreads.

## DISORGANIZATION

The stage called *disorganization* is a highly traumatic period for virtually everyone who experiences it. It is typically, although not universally, heralded by intense confusion, despair, and anxiety, as coping mechanisms patients invoked during the stage of awareness begin to crumble. During this stage, patients finally realize, often with a sudden shock of conviction, that something really is wrong—a realization beyond any possibility for rationalization or denial. It is no longer possible to deny or hope the problem will somehow disappear. The EKG is confirmatory. It *is* a heart attack. A second HIV antibody test comes back positive. It *is* an HIV infection. In some patients, the moment of truth comes long before official pronouncements or confirmatory laboratory tests. For others, it may be forestalled, as patients continue to protest even in the face of hard evidence, "That just *can't* be right!" When the realization occurs, however, a profound disruption in functioning results. Suddenly, everything has changed, leaving patients feeling overwhelmed, powerless, helpless, and shattered. Hopes, dreams, plans for the future may no longer pertain. Important relationships are suddenly altered. Patients' relationship to their own *body* is altered dramatically. Above all, patients now experience a *shattering of omnipotence.*

When people find it impossible to deny any longer that something is seriously wrong, a universal human defense is demolished—the magical belief, "It could never happen to me." Disease, disfigurement, death—these things happen to *someone else, not to me.* Human hubris and self-deception are involved, yet we choose this mindset, as long as we remain healthy. Indeed, the deception seems to be almost integral to normal functioning, and when this defense goes, an individual's reality changes radically. One reason, we believe, physicians and other caretakers often shun dying patients has to do with this defense. The undisputable *truth* of death is embodied too vividly in the sight of a suffering, terminal patient. The most dedicated among us may be tempted to back away to preserve *our* illusion of omnipotence.

During this stage, patients feel cut off, and indeed they are. Sick people are severed from all their usual connections to everyday life—schedules, habits, activities, friends, family, and work as well as hobbies, TV shows, favorite pipes, coffee mugs, and slippers. They are trundled down tiled corridors through doors that say NO ADMITTANCE. Naked, they are dressed in a hospital gown and deposited in an unfamiliar hospital bed, dependent on anonymous, if well-intentioned, strangers. No wonder they feel isolated, depressed, and demoralized—cut off not only from their routine and people, but from their very sense of self. There are accompanying distortions in thinking that occur during this stage—increasingly idiosyncratic, superstitious, and self-centered preoccupations that ill people abhor, yet cannot help. Strangely, perhaps, there is often guilt. Many patients believe at some level that their illness is a punishment for some transgression. For others, illness invokes a sense of helpless rage. Like Job, they ask bitterly, "Why me?"

That this period of crisis is profoundly painful for patients should be obvious. To be effective, physicians must have empathy for the turmoil their patients are suffering. They must be able to reach out across that chasm of terror, isolation, and loneliness as best they can. To do this, they have to have done some serious introspecting of their own and come to some inner peace about their own mortality. If they have not, they will back away defensively just when their patients need them most. Physicians should also recognize that, although no patient would ever invite such a crisis, the radical introspection it forces on a person can lead to increased wisdom and new life perspectives. Illness always seems to yield a bitter harvest, but sometimes it bears unanticipated fruit—the opportunity to expand as a person, to change, and to grow.

During the stage of disorganization, some people progress to death rapidly. Many more, mercifully, go on to recovery. Usually they, too, try to "forget," but really there can be no forgetting. Once people have been seriously ill, they *have* changed. A man who has had a heart attack is not the same man who has *not* had a heart attack. His cardiac enzymes may be back to normal. His EKG may be unremarkable. He may take up jogging and achieve a robust new sense of health. Whatever he does or does not do; however, he is, forever after, a man who has had a heart attack. In life, the moving hand does, indeed, write. Whatever the eventual outcome of a specific illness, that hand moves continuously onward. A heart attack or a bout with cancer can never be undone, washed out, canceled from memory. We can excise a tumor from a person's body, but we cannot abate the meaning of that experience from a patient's life. Above all, we believe the shattering of omnipotence changes a person from then on. Of course, the terror recedes and the defenses return, but at some level people who have been seriously ill have seen their own mortality. These people are altered—wise on occasion, often not—but not the same. By the very nature of their work, a similar transformation also occurs in most doctors.

## REORGANIZATION

Although the reality of illness seems overwhelming at first—imagine what it would be like to suddenly have cancer—the stage of disorganization is usually surprisingly brief. Somehow, the unbearable is borne; the unthinkable is assimilated—and all this with an alacrity that is sometimes astonishing. At some point, and usually sooner than later, ill people begin to accept the reality of their disease and to grasp the changes it has wrought, the tasks in the future that must be faced. Ill people begin to acknowledge, in one form or another, that the illness is no longer something foreign that has happened to them. Rather, they realize, "It is me. I have not been *attacked* by diabetes, I am a person *with* diabetes." Typically, patients' emergence from disorganization into reorganization is heralded by statements such as: "You've got to go on" or "You can't lay around feeling sorry for yourself forever" or "What's done is done; you've got to accept it and move on." These and similar expressions convey two essential features of the stage of reorganization: (1) the *recognition* that one cannot stop time or turn back the clock ("You have to go on") and (2) *acceptance* (patients no longer fight or deny the reality of their condition).

For patients and their families, the reorganization phase is the most important part of the illness. For example, if you were to ask a woman who has undergone a radical mastectomy for breast cancer to describe her experience, chances are she would dwell primarily on concerns that pertain to the reorganization phase—living with the disfigurement, the fears of recurrence, worries about the reaction of her husband, where to get mastectomy brassieres—all the things that would matter to any woman facing life with a recent diagnosis of cancer and the hasty amputation of one of her breasts. Contrast this picture, however, with what her *physician* would likely say were *he* asked to describe Mrs. Smith's bout with breast cancer. Very likely, he would launch into a discussion of diagnosis, staging, pathology reports, questions of radiation therapy versus chemotherapy, and whether a mastectomy or a lumpectomy was indicated. This is perfectly understandable. Such technical considerations are a large part of what every physician thinks about and does. Yet, we can also see the physician's concerns are very much out of harmony with his patient's. In contrast to her concerns, most of which have to do with the phase of reorganization, the physician is concerned primarily with the disorganization phase of illness. Clearly, this can be a serious problem. From the outset of their education, medical students are exposed almost exclusively to people in the stage of disorganization—hospitalized patients who are in the most acute stages of illness. As soon as patients are stable enough to leave the hospital, they are discharged from students' care and, all too often, from students' mind. Experienced physicians in primary care who see such patients year after year know reality is far different; but, young physicians in training, prior to entering outpatient clinical care, tend to view the experience of illness and the scope of their responsibilities as being limited to the phase of disorganization. Nothing could be more misleading because, from patients' perspectives and their families', when the time for discharge from the hospital arrives, the illness process has barely just *begun*.

A better understanding of what patients face during reorganization is far from trivial. It is here that physicians can often make a real difference. This phase contains great opportunities for growth, increased wisdom, a deeper sense of love, and enhanced spiritual meaning. It also contains the equally real potential for human failure. Patients may give up, withdraw, and become embittered and defeated for the rest of their life.

We are all moved by sagas of heroism, stamina, and grace displayed by the gravely ill. Helen Keller's courage has moved people for generations and will doubtless continue to do so. We all admire the rectitude and forbearance of Franklin Delano Roosevelt, who conducted the presidency from his wheelchair. Lou Gehrig died of amyotrophic lateral sclerosis (since then called Lou Gehrig's disease), but the nation remembers him most for the dignity he displayed to the very end. David Rosen has multiple sclerosis, but he does not let his illness define him. In fact, he continues to see patients (albeit less than before) and he has even become a comedian (see his YouTube video *Dr. Nada, Live at the Tiny Tavern*)[3].

In contrast, we are considerably less comfortable with reorganization's darker side. Many physicians feel highly uncomfortable when confronted by patients who *fail* to "get better," "take care of themselves," or "do their part." Permit an example: A formerly successful businessman has a myocardial infarction and then becomes a "cardiac cripple." A year later, his myocardium has mended, but he has resigned his employment and lives on disability insurance. His wife is distraught and on the verge of divorcing him because of his brooding self-preoccupation and refusal to initiate any sexual activity whatsoever. He has given up all hobbies, sports, and interests. Most days he just sits, watches television, and broods. He laments, with melancholic self-pity, that his life is "over." Initially, perhaps, a physician has sympathy for such a patient. She may exhort him to try harder, reminding him that the prognosis is much better than he seems to believe. Sooner or later, though, the physician is apt to grow weary and defeated, and get "turned off" by this patient's stonewalling and ultimate failure to surmount his illness and go on with life. Finally, such patients get labeled. They are called "chronics," or "psych cases." These cruel and casually misapplied epithets refer, of course, to human beings, and their use should always be discouraged. When they are used in this context, however, the doctor is communicating something very specific. She is saying, "I can't stand the sight of helplessness, passivity, dependence, depression, and giving up. These are all experiences I would fight in myself and would dread ever succumbing to. Therefore, when I see a patient succumbing to them, I feel threatened and I experience revulsion."

Many factors ultimately determine whether patients grow or regress during this stage: (1) the patient's personality and previous experience with illness and doctors, (2) the meaning of the illness to the patient, (3) the patient's support system, (4) the patient's environment, (5) the severity and nature of the disease process (eg, a malignant and disfiguring illness may be especially devastating), and (6) the effectiveness of medical care, including that given by the patient's doctor.

Sometimes, it is true, we doctors have a perception of ourselves that is grandiose and inflated. Here, however, the problem is actually the opposite: For many of us, it is difficult to acknowledge that we matter so much. Patients who are brave, dignified, and successful are obviously going to be easier for us to deal with than those who are frightened, regressed, angry, and inconsolable. Yet, the latter comprise many of our patients. They need us, too. Sometimes they need us the most of all. Could it be that our "cardiac cripple" might have been helped, might *still* be helped, by a physician who took the time—not to give more lectures of stiff-upper-lip pep talks, but to form an empathic alliance in which the patient felt supported and understood? Perhaps with such an alliance he still might feel safe enough to face what frightens him. Possibly. We should also consider the worst. It is possible that this patient, even with the best of support from his physician, will *still* fail to bounce back. These depressing outcomes can and do occur in medicine. All the time. Even with this, is he our patient any the less? Does he need us any the less? To the contrary, it is this patient who needs us most. Isolated, rigid, unable to change, such patients experience profound loneliness and suffering. Eventually they drive everyone away, psychologically if not figuratively. They grow to be shunned by society and are held in contempt (something they are aware of). Perhaps *only* a physician can transcend these prejudices and manage to view the suffering patient in an accepting and nonjudgmental manner. Surely the patient is in pain. Even if we cannot cure him of the corrosive nihilism that is eating away at his soul, we can still soothe him. We can reassure him we will not abandon him. As doctors, we can attempt as best we can to ease his pain and suffering—one of our most ancient and fundamental responsibilities.

In closing this section, we wish to repeat what we said earlier: This view of illness as a developmental process is only a model. Like any model, it can be useful if it provides a foundation for increased conceptual clarity and understanding. It can remain useful as long as it remains heuristic and is not applied mindlessly, uncritically. Unfortunately, models have a considerable tendency to degenerate into nostrums and "gospel truths," at which point they lose their usefulness. The advantage of viewing illness as development, as long as we heed our previous warning, may be twofold. First, modern medicine tends to forget people are part of a rich and complicated life setting, a context in which all of them fall ill. Doctors trained in contemporary medical institutions all too often seem to regard the world as though it were a huge admissions area, depositing endless legions of sick people at the physician's doorstep to be examined and studied. Actually, doctors and hospitals are threads woven through the fabric of a person's experience, not the warp and weft of life itself. Second, emphasizing illness as development does draw our attention to another neglected area—the importance of the physician *throughout* a patient's illness. In an earlier era, doctors had come to think of themselves as responsible for patients only during the most acute phase of illness—a problem we discussed previously. Graduate medical education has transitioned to increased teaching in ambulatory care settings to train future physicians adequately. This is crucial given the bulk of our patients are people with life-long disease. The afflictions may vary—from arthritis to diabetes, from heart disease to schizophrenia. What they all have in common is that they do not go away. By thinking of illness as development, it may be easier for doctors to begin to understand what it would be like to be someone with a chronic illness, a life-long illness—what it would really mean to walk in that person's shoes, not for a few yards or quarter of a mile, but for the distance, mile upon mile, year stretching into year. We doctors are needed along that pathway, too.

## THE EXPERIENCES OF ILLNESS DEPENDS ON WHO THE PERSON IS

In large measure, the experience of illness depends on who the person is. It is for this reason we must heed our patients' personality and coping styles, not simply because we wish to psychologize. How individuals handle being sick reflects their attitudes, defenses, strengths, weaknesses, and philosophy of life. If the sick person is a "fighter," for example, one who always seems to bounce back from adversity, this style may well predict how she will cope with serious illness. A superb example of such a fighter is depicted in *Heartsounds* by Martha Weinman Lear[4]. This book is a very moving account of a doctor's own cardiac illness as it progresses through acute and chronic stages and finally ends in death. The book was written by his wife, with much input from the physician himself, and maintains an intensely personal tone throughout. It is eminently readable and richly instructive, a book difficult to put down once you begin. The account begins with Dr. Harold Lear's first heart attack and his initial adjustment to that sudden illness. Eventually, he undergoes open-heart surgery and, as a result, succumbs tragically to organic brain damage. Yet, right up to his death he remains a fighter. His will to live is truly astounding and inspiring.

Dr. Lear expresses how he felt when he realized modern technological medicine had nothing to offer him and he was going to die. His reflections also illustrate a positive outcome in the transition from disorganization to reorganization. He faces his reality, but he does not give up:

> I am not losing hope . . . . I know I'm not going to get any better. That's hard to take. What always helped me in the past was thinking, later I'll be better. I don't think that any more—wiping his eyes—but I'm not giving up. I'm simply accepting my realities. I may challenge them sporadically, but my denial is much less now. The closer people can be to their realities, the better off they are.
>
> The paradox is that in many ways I'm happier now than I've ever been. I never thought about how I might cope with sickness. I was the doctor. Now I look back at all these things that happened to me, emerging from these experiences with holes in my head, and I wonder how I was able to cope. What was there in me that allowed me to survive as well as I did emotionally? Why aren't I in a deep depression? I don't

know. I guess it's still my father. "You've got to make the best of it." That's what he always told me. And I try to, and I'll never give up. (ref. 4, p. 371)

The profound, critical importance of this—not giving up—is also expressed by the young physician who cared for Harold Lear during the last months of his life. Dr. Fried gave this eulogy at Dr. Lear's funeral:

> Since the way a man dies, just as the way he lives, is often a solid measure of his spirit, it is appropriate that we share perceptions of his very last days .... Harold Lear was a physician who understood every detail of his pathology and prognosis. He knew exactly the conditions of battle, he was not awed, and he fought like hell. (ref. 4, p. 498)

It is clear that Dr. Fried fought like hell, too. Like his physician–patient, Dr. Fried also did not give up. Along with Dr. Lear's own family, the young physician stood by him with unwavering support.

Dr. Lear wanted *Heartsounds* to be written because he felt that if physicians knew what it is really like to be profoundly ill they would treat their patients far differently, with much greater sensitivity and empathy, perhaps also with more courage and a sense of pride and hope. Read it. We think you will agree.

Elsewhere in the book, Lear's wife cries out in consternation, lamenting a physician who, she felt, abandoned her husband at a critical point in his care. He is referred to as Moses, or Moe, in the text, and in the passage below, she castigates him for transferring her husband's care to his younger associate just when the going got rough:

> You do not do such a thing, Moses, to such a patient who comes to you at such a time, humbled by disease. You perhaps have never been deeply and chronically ill; you perhaps do not know from within how sickness humbles—how it clouds and corrodes and befouls the sense of self. I do not know why this should be so, that physical disease plays such cruel vanquishing tricks upon the ego, even the sturdiest ego, given time enough. But I have seen it happen here, to this fine strong man, and I have read a bit about such things and I know that this is classic in long chronic disease; this is what the failures of the body do unerringly to the soul. And I know this much, Moses, surely you know it too. And you are neither an unkind nor an uncaring man. So why do you reject him now, when his ego is so fragile? Could it be that yours is not fragile enough? Too thick a hide, eh? Or that you are angry at this sick patient for remaining so intransigently sick? Or—this being my darkest suspicion—that you can do nothing more for him and so choose, in subliminal ways, to wash your hands? Not that I wish illness upon you, Moses, may you never have illness, but perhaps it would teach doctors something they do not know. Or know only theoretically, which is not enough. Perhaps there should be a way to induce illness, pseudo-illness, something dreadful but safe, with clear parameters, that would last, say, for a year and wreak all due havoc upon the body and spirit before it disappeared. A required course at all medical schools; no one graduates without two consecutive semesters of chronic, debilitating sickness. What do

you think, Moe, old friend, old eminence: would that make better doctors? (ref. 4, pp. 272–273)

Mrs. Lear is obviously very angry, and understandably so, but she raises a key question: What enabled Dr. Fried to care and remain attached when Moses could not? She ventures a plausible guess: Moe fled not because he was so callous, but because Lear's dying hurt too much. Although her anger at Moe is understandable, we should not follow suit. Instead, we should try to understand. It is difficult to remain committed to suffering, dying patients, especially when they are doctors like ourselves. For Moe, older and more vulnerable, it might have been too much like looking in a mirror. Moe, in fact, attended the funeral visibly in pain. This was not the act of a cold and indifferent man. Like Chiron, of Greek legend, Moe had been wounded—a wounded healer.

Dr. Lear's heroism is inspiring. Yet we must also be prepared for patients who respond very differently—who regress, fall apart, give up. These people, too, have their reasons. No one chooses to fail consciously, and often there are discernible reasons why people do. How would Dr. Lear have fared, for instance, without his wife's tremendous love and support? Our empathy must go out all the more to those patients who are not so brave, who are "difficult" or "weak." Doctors are often surprisingly, and disturbingly, angered by these so-called "problem patients." We believe part of the difficulty may come from the physician's own fears of regressing and losing control. Few prospects frighten doctors more.

We have been talking, of course, about the pivotal importance of hope. Over and over, our patients teach us that hope is crucial and sometimes highly predictive of prognosis as well. We cannot measure hope, unfortunately, the way we can stage lymphomas; yet, its vicissitudes are just as important and its effects just as powerful. With relentless regularity, patients who give up deteriorate quickly. The phenomenon cannot be explained by levels of organ impairment alone. The matter is still more complex: Just as the physically afflicted go downhill after they give up, somatic illness itself is often heralded by circumstances in life in which a physically healthy person gives up hope. This surrender can take many forms. A classic one is severe grief. It is well illustrated by the case of a woman we shall simply call Mrs. Smith. The story begins with the husband.

Mr. Smith, a 68-year-old man with metastatic bronchogenic carcinoma, was admitted to the hospital because of marked difficulty breathing. Examination disclosed large bilateral pleural effusions. Mrs. Smith was 67 years old and required daily insulin for her diabetes. During Mr. Smith's hospitalization, she was constantly at his bedside, day and night. On the third hospital day, Mr. Smith began coughing up massive amounts of blood and died. Mrs. Smith was comforted briefly and was then asked to give permission for the autopsy. She assented. The busy physician in charge of the case then had no further contact with Mrs. Smith, nor did he expect to. Ten days later, Mrs. Smith was back all too forcefully. She came in comatose; her diagnosis: severe diabetic ketoacidosis. With rapid and appropriate management, she soon regained consciousness. When queried about what had transpired, she lucidly described a deep feeling of exhaustion. She just could not muster the energy to give herself her insulin injections after her husband's death. Yes, she said she understood the consequences of this inaction, but had felt totally paralyzed and inert.

Throughout the course of her hospitalizations, with the assistance of a sensitive medical student, she began to express her profound sorrow and sense of loss since her husband's death. When she was discharged, she still grieved but was able to manage her insulin and diet once again. In a real sense, helping her to begin the grief process permitted her to resume control over her diabetes and her life.

Engel also illustrates the giving-up response dramatically in his paper, "Giving-up/Given-up Complex[5]":

This concerns a couple, Charlie and Josephine, who had been inseparable companions for 13 years. In a senseless act of violence Charlie, in full view of Josephine, was shot and killed in a melee with the police. Josephine first stood motionless, then slowly approached his prostrate form, sunk to her knees, and silently rested her head on the dead and bloody body. Concerned persons attempted to help her away, but she refused to move. Hoping she would soon surmount her overwhelming grief, they let her be. But she never rose again; in 15 minutes she was dead.

Now the remarkable part of the story is that Charlie and Josephine were llamas in the zoo! They had escaped from their pen during a snow storm and Charlie, a mean animal to begin with, was shot when he proved unmanageable. I was able to establish from the zoo keeper that to all intents and purposes Josephine had been normally frisky and healthy right up to the moment of the tragic event. No autopsy was performed, so we can go no further in explaining the death. (ref. 5, pp. 293–300).

Engel cites this example not simply for drama, but also to underscore the fact that we are dealing with an evolutionarily deep, essentially mammalian phenomenon. Devastating, even fatal grief is not simply a quirk of "neurotic" and "oversensitive" human beings; attachment is rooted in biology, and loss really can break a heart and end a life.

Schmale[6] and Engel[5] outline five characteristics of a condition they call the "giving-up/given-up" complex, which seems to be associated with the onset of illness: (1) feelings of helplessness and/or hopelessness; (2) a depreciated self-image; (3) a loss of pleasure and meaning normally derived from important relationships and roles in life; (4) a disrupted sense of the vital continuity in one's life that links past, present, and future; and (5) a reactivation of memories of earlier periods of giving up. It seems to constitute a psychological state in which vulnerability to pathogenic factors is increased.

The myriad ways in which people respond to illness are naturally as varied as people are themselves. Although it is useful to delineate some general principles about how patients respond to illness, people are just too rich, complex, and innately resilient to fit into any neat schemata. Generalities help but do not suffice when we face the person in that bed who is sick and needs our help.

To assist our patients as individuals is possible. Although people cannot be categorized neatly, approaches to understanding people can. A few of the important ones are learning about patients' personality structure or style, their usual coping mechanisms, the adaptive and maladaptive experiences in their life, their past experiences with illness, their family relationships and circumstances, and their personal attitudes. The superordinating principle is to attempt to understand each person as a unique individual;

this is not impossible. Given the chance to talk about themselves, provided by the patient-centered interview approach described in Chapter 5, they usually tell you what is important about themselves, and these disclosures have a value that goes far beyond establishing rapport. If you can find out from your patients who they are and who they have been, you will have a good chance to know who they are about to be—and you do not have to be a genius. They will tell you, if only you will listen! And watch! And feel! This knowledge obviously has immediate and compelling relevance to one's treatment approach, one's style of supporting your patients' own strengths, and one's sense of the maladaptive behaviors to look for in particular patients. Recall Ms. Johnson (Johnnie) and Mr. Glover in Chapters 1 and 2.

## CHALLENGES OF ILLNESS

Illness—any illness—disrupts. But, as we have seen in Dr. Rosen's case, it can be the seed of creative change. Illness poses serious and sometimes horrendous challenges. Some of these have been described by Moos and Tsu.[7] The list is vivid, but we should heed it for it is also very accurate, although inevitably incomplete.

1. *Dealing with pain, discomfort, and incapacitation*: These are a part of every illness. The amount of pain and its intensity vary with each patient. All pain is real, and understanding patients' perception of their pain is critical to effective care. Also, understanding patients' view of their illness and the accompanying incapacitation or disability are essential to helping each one recover from acute illness or to accept limitations in function associated with chronic illness.
2. *Dealing with the problems posed by treatment procedures themselves* and the actual hospital environment (eg, the special concerns imposed by invasive diagnostic tests and by the ICU or CCU experience): Patients undergoing technical procedures and treatments with real risks and in strange hospital environments cry out for helpful information, understanding, and human support.
3. *Developing positive relationships with caregivers*: For example, dealing with conflicting information, staff styles, and covert and overt disagreements can not only be merely bothersome, but also terrifying. To take a common example, many patients find it difficult to engage their physicians in a true partnership, one in which patients feel their preferences about treatment are respected and heeded. Breakdowns in the therapeutic relationship may arise from shortcomings on either side of that critical dyad. Yet, when these occur, it is all too tempting for doctors to blame their patients, attributing the patients' apparent intransigence to "neurosis" or a bad attitude. Sometimes, physicians retaliate; ironically, the "punishment" is occasionally a psychiatry consult. In contrast, astute clinicians strive continually to monitor and understand their own reactions to their patients. There is actually a gold mine of information about difficulties patients are having—not the frustration that is so often perceived. Some patients, of course, do have difficult and even contratherapeutic character styles. They cannot help it, and such patients challenge the wisest, kindest, cleverest, and most tolerant among us. How ironic that these very people are so typically thrust on impressionable young students and house officers as their first

learning cases! Yet, the rewards of making a difference in the lives of such people—even a small one—can be immeasurable. More often than one might think, students turn out to be the very best physicians for these "impossible patients" whom others have written off.

4. *Dealing with upsetting feelings*: As great as the physical discomfort can be, the mental pain of illness is often even worse. Patients suffer feelings of grief over physical loss or incapacitation, apprehension about the future, self-blame, failure, and isolation from people who are healthy. Such feelings are always difficult. Nor is the absence of feeling in patients at all reassuring. Most likely, they are denying, failing to deal with the realities they face. Some degree of denial is inevitable and, in fact, healthy ("I know I'll come through; my surgeon's the greatest!"). Yet all too often we see something palpably different from healthy denial: the suffering patient who withdraws, refuses to comply or perhaps drinks, and ultimately gives up all feelings of connectedness and hope. Such despair, and it is common, militates against natural healing processes. For physicians true to their profession, the restoration of hope to such patients should be paramount.

5. *Maintaining an acceptable self-image*: We all need a sense of independence, integrity of identity, and autonomy in life. Illness, with its inevitable tug toward regression and dependence, can be devastating. To survive is one thing; to be truly alive, we must preserve our sense of self-worth. Illness can challenge this in ways that are utterly malicious. Consider the patient whose face is burned or whose breast has been amputated or whose testicles have been removed. These are visible kinds of insult. Think of a college professor with dementia who cannot remember the date. The assault on one's self-esteem can be savage, deeply poignant, and bitterly unfair.

6. *Preserving satisfying relationships with family, friends, and coworkers*: Beyond the figurative physical separation caused by illness and hospitalization, being sick effects subtler forms of alienation. Almost universally, an emotional separation from other people sets in as well. An invisible yet impenetrable barrier separates the sick from the well—indeed, the sick person from herself. As doctors, we can reach out and ease the loneliness, but we cannot take it away. Sick people face their fate, in some ways, alone. We can help more by empathizing with this truth than by trying to be facile and denying it. Illness is always a harbinger of life's inevitable experience—death itself—and this we all will face, and face alone.

## COPING

When people become ill, they must adapt, for better or worse. Those who love and depend on them must also adjust. No one welcomes such change. It is simply inescapable. Therefore major illness poses a serious, totally uninvited developmental crisis: One's dreams, self-image, and plans must all be reconsidered or even abandoned. It is no small undertaking.

The ability of patients and their families to cope with this challenge determines not only the course of the illness itself, but also the quality of life that follows. Helping to maximize our patients' success in this momentous struggle is also part of our responsibility as doctors. Attempts by physicians to deny this are as common as they are absurd, yet we believe such denials are not born of callousness, but from bewilderment. Most physicians have not been schooled during their education to help their patients in just these ways. Within medical education, the lack of such a perspective remains a glaring deficiency, although one that is being addressed increasingly. There is much cause for optimism. Yet, many students would add, much potential for rhetoric, moralizing, and vagueness lurks here. Treating the whole patient sounds fine, but how? In a real sense, this entire book evolved as a response to just this question: But how? How, without mysticism, clichés, or platitudes, can we take care of the total human being?

You must indulge us here and permit a brief explanation of what is, essentially, a teaching problem. We explicate it at this point because we believe clarification will help students to understand better the dilemmas faced by those who wish to teach this broad perspective of patient care. Essentially, the risks in teaching this subject run to unhelpful pigeonholing at one extreme and excessive vagueness and ambiguity at the other. All students, no doubt, have encountered educators who commit one error or the other, perhaps even both. Yet, how to convey this material effectively is not so obvious or easy, especially when confronted with a subject as complicated as a human being. Discussions of patient "types," "classic" defenses, and "typical" problems are rife in the literature. They offer the allure of apparent neatness and order—"the seven patient types"—and even lists to be committed to memory. Patients, by their sheer diversity, outfox us, however. Inevitably they wiggle free from our neat pigeonholes. At the other extreme, generalizing about caring for the "whole person" without substantiating it in practice does not help either. Such admonitions arm students with little that is applicable or useful, full as they may be of indisputably noble sentiments. For a comprehensive guide to caring for the whole person, to include both patient and clinician, please avail yourself to Dr. David Kopacz's *Re-humanizing Medicine*[8].

In what follows, we offer some frameworks and categories, maybe even a pigeonhole or two. You must remember we are providing tools for understanding, not conceptual chains and shackles. Bear in mind that these concepts, like all tools, are there to help us understand our patients better, not to carve them up into some predetermined shape. These frameworks within the limits imposed by individual complexity and sheer variety offer doctors some handles—attitudes and approaches that may ease the suffering our patients so often endure. The concept of "coping with illness," no matter how acute or cataclysmic, is always, in some way and to some extent, made to mesh with the basic and enduring themes of a patient's life. Put another way: In time, illness becomes an integrated part of the process of that person's life. How we manage the vicissitudes of that process can be critical in a patient's life—for good or ill.

Ways of coping are sometimes called *defense mechanisms*. We prefer the less glamorous term because it emphasizes the universality and often nonpathological nature of these mechanisms. When threatened, we all experience anxiety and try to reduce it. To do this, typically we invoke the mental and physical tricks that have worked in the past. For example, the intellectual attempts to cope by reasoning, the athlete by "working out," and so on—if, of course, one can perform such tasks, for illness often plays cruel tricks. Typically, coping mechanisms contain within them a considerable range of extremes and can be understood from the perspective of dichotomies. Here are some of the more common ones:

*Inward turning versus outward turning*: Some people seem to retreat "inside" when sick; others seek increased interaction with friends, family, and even strangers.

*Organized versus disorganized*: Some gain strength by focusing on details, order, and regularity; others abandon efforts to keep things "straight" and in order.

*Confrontation versus avoidance*: Some need "to know" and seem most comfortable when they are kept fully informed of all aspects of their situation; others seem to avoid knowing (at lease consciously) and may "forget" or deny truths.

*Dominant versus submissive*: In the face of illness, some people find it helpful to maximize their control and mastery over as many areas of their lives as they can; others regress and yearn for others to "take over for a while."

*Creativity versus stagnation*: Do what you have always wanted to do. Don't let illness disable you; rather, let it enable you. Writing *Transforming Depression: Healing the Soul through Creativity*[9] helped David to deal with his reactive depression after a divorce.

Several observations must be made here. These guidelines do have important implications for caring for patients: To which patient do we tell the bold truth? Who needs a lot of control over his or her own treatment? Who requires that we take over? Who needs to be comforted? Who needs to be left alone? Our ability to identify these trends correctly in our patients can enhance their comfort and, occasionally, head off disaster. Remember also, though, they are just trends. In truth, we feel both ways at different times, perhaps even at the same time. The stoic who says, "Tell it like it is," may nonetheless experience terrible dread. The woman who says, "Leave me alone," may yet long for closeness and comfort. We must learn to diagnose changing trends and watch for shifting vectors of these polarities over time. Never assume patients remain fixed along this continuation.

It should also be clear that such coping mechanisms are not pathological per se. They can be, of course, but often the trick for skilled clinicians involves helping patients use the coping methods they already have to their best advantage: Allow Mr. Adams to be involved with decisions regarding his treatment; let Mrs. Jones leave matters "in your hands, doctor."

Above all, help patients not to give up. Moos and Tsu[7] have identified several indicators that patients are coping effectively with their illness. These generally include minimizing or even denying the seriousness of the illness; seeking relevant information, particularly about the illness and the medical procedures or interventions that will affect them; seeking reassurance and emotional support; setting limited yet realistic and concrete goals; rehearsing alternative outcomes; and, last but not least, seeking to derive new purpose, meaning, and direction in life despite the illness experience. Conversely, the absence of these signs should be regarded as ominous.

This, of course, does not exhaust the repertoire of coping styles and skills in our patients, but it hopefully provides guideposts. Pay attention to the "track record." The way people have coped with other serious stressors in their life is an excellent predictor of how they will cope now. No pat generalizations about the "ulcer personality" or "migraine personality" can replace a thorough understanding of how any particular patient is apt to react when frightened, uncertain, and in pain.

The following case exemplifies how recognition and understanding of coping styles can contribute to improved patient care:

> Ms. S, a 26-year-old woman, was admitted to the hospital because of acute bacterial endocarditis. Although this was her second hospitalization for the same condition, she seemed guarded and distrustful, able to confide only in one particular nurse and her own personal attending physician. For the rest of the staff, she remained very aloof. It would have been tempting for the rest of the staff to dismiss her—"an unappreciative patient"—but they did not. For all her aloofness, Ms. S was overheard repeatedly expressing anguished concerns that she "look well" for her boyfriend. She was keenly aware of his visits and became visibly distraught when he failed to appear.
>
> As the staff accepted and did not reject or overpersonalize her discomfort with strangers, it became easier for them to tolerate her tendency toward emotional distance. Yet, they did not abandon her in response to this. Instead, the staff made a special effort to provide regular, consistent people to work with her. Consistency seemed important, and trust, though hard won, continued to be a goal the staff had while working with this patient. Respecting her need for distance did not, consequently, become carte blanche for her caretakers to abdicate responsibility for this woman.
>
> Especially, the staff wanted to do something about her obviously agonizing dread that she might lose her boyfriend. He was strongly encouraged to visit predictably. The staff encouraged him to discuss plans for their future together—one beyond her illness. The realistically predictable course of the illness and its possible complications were reviewed with the patient exactingly. Every attempt was made to dispel frightening distortions that she harbored about a bleak future and, most especially, her fears her illness would destroy her relationship with her boyfriend beyond salvageability.
>
> Never did she become overtly tearful or emotionally effusive. The staff was able to appreciate that this was her way of coping. In fact, when she did become visibly upset, she asked to be "left alone." Even her few select confidants on the staff were not welcome at such times. When she was highly distressed she would withdraw into a flurry of "housekeeping." She would tidy her hospital room, for example, in a meticulous, yet driven and stereotyped fashion. The staff saw this for what it was—not "pathology," but this particular woman's inevitable attempt to cope with the threat of possible loss and emotional chaos by maintaining a tight web of superficial control as best she could. This was *her* way. The staff was sensitive and wise enough to understand and accept she preferred it to "our way."
>
> During the hospitalization, she was immensely comforted and helped. Imagine how different the outcome might have been if the staff had insisted that she "open up" and do it "our way"—or worse—had simply written her off as too remote and distant to be bothered with at all.

## "PROBLEM PATIENTS"

No one can be long in a hospital or clinic without learning that some persons are labeled "problem patients." Nevertheless, we discourage reductionistic, cookbook typologies that promise magical techniques for approaching "the seven kinds of problem patients." Closer scrutiny usually reveals these are patients who are coping with their illness in ways the doctor does not approve or understand—not some candidates for pigeonholes or recipes of patient "types." The coping styles of such patients often serve these patients and their families well, but they collide with hospital routine, orderly operation, and, above all, doctors' own beliefs about how a sick person should act and behave. When this occurs, sparks fly, and we have, as often as not, "a problem patient." Yet, it is useful to step back at such times and ask: Why is the patient behaving this way? From his perspective, there must be a reason. Above all, it is always worth asking: Does this patient's behavior disrupt him or does it nettle us and our own values? Is this the actual problem that leads us to feel such a patient is "sabotaging" the treatment and fighting against the therapy? More often than not, such a query leads to an obvious, yet important recognition. These patients are not usually fighting what is "good" for them; they simply have an entirely different view of what this "good" might be.

Kleinman, Eisenberg, and Good[10] have called this the problem of discrepant "explanatory models." An awareness of this extremely common phenomenon is important. It leads to a reduction in futile, angry finger-pointing and encourages in its place an open-minded inquiry about where the discrepancy lies. This is well illustrated by these authors' own clinical vignette from their article in *Annals of Internal Medicine*:

> Mrs. F. is a 60 year old white Protestant grandmother who is recovering on one of the medical wards from pulmonary edema, atherosclerotic cardiovascular disease, and chronic congestive heart failure. Her behavior in the recovery phase of her illness is described as strange and annoying by the house staff and nurses. While her cardiac status has greatly improved and she has become virtually asymptomatic, she nevertheless repeatedly induces vomiting and urinates frequently into her bed. And she becomes very angry when told to stop. Psychiatric consultation is quickly requested. Review of her lengthy medical record reveals nothing about the personal significance of this bizarre behavior. When queried about it, however, and encouraged to explain why she is doing what she is, her response is most revealing. She begins by reminding the doctor that she is the wife and daughter of plumbers.
>
> Furthermore, she reminds the consultant that she was told that she had "water in the lungs." She goes on to report that her understanding of anatomy is equally hydraulic: The human body has a chest hooked up to two pipes—namely, the mouth and the urethra. Consequently, she has been trying to be helpful by removing as much water from her chest as possible through self-induced vomiting and frequent urination. She analogizes the latter to the work of the "water pills" that she is taking that, indeed, the doctors told her were for getting rid of the water in her chest. Logic is logic! She concludes: "I can't understand why people are angry at me." After appropriate explanations, along with diagrams, she was eventually able to understand that the "plumbing" of the body was quite different from her

conception. Her unusual behavior ended at that time. A "problem patient" also vanished (ref. 10, pp. 251–258).

Certainly, patients can be obnoxious and act irrational, but usually, with effort, we can understand their "folly." Keep in mind that, as humans, we are all highly diverse and endlessly creative beings, always looking for ways to turn difficult events to our own uses, even when the events are profound disruptions, such as illness. Apart from the fact that certain kinds of psychological situations seem to predispose people to illness onset, the illness itself can—and indeed must—be integrated into a person's life. Often this unappreciated creativity, in which patients turn undesirable afflictions into avenues to achieve desirable ends, is pejoratively labeled "secondary gain." However, it is more complex than that. Patients do learn the ropes and often make almost exasperating use of the bureaucratic and institutional red tape we have created in the first place. It is easy to label such people pejoratively as "manipulators." A few are, but more are not. They are adapting creatively—albeit with sometimes pungent irony—to the circumstances we have placed in their path. "Compensation medicine" is fraught with these issues, and there are a host of publications about the "accident process" and the "illness process." Yet, when we confront such apparent monsters as the "compensation patient," we should not, as Dr. Frankenstein did, forget too quickly who actually yanked the lever on the transformer that supplied the juice. In fact, studies of such patients usually show they are behaving in ways entirely consistent with their prior life experience. They are coping as life and the system have taught them to cope. We can intervene effectively, but not if we condemn hastily. If you search in such patients' behavior for what is *creative* and even ingenious, you will usually find it. This is a general principle, of which the so-called "compensation neurotic" is only an extreme instance. Most "problem patients" are coping with problems. Most irrational behavior turns out to make sense, given patients' experiences and beliefs. Their attempts are usually efforts at self-cure—self-healing attempts to understand and improve aspects of life that are unsatisfactory, painful, and frightening. These attempts are not always rational or wise, but as caretakers we cannot assist if we condemn before we attempt to understand.

## REFERENCES

1. Nasim M, Becerra L, Borsook D. Migraine: maladaptive brain responses to stress. *Headache.* 2012;52 (2):102–106.
2. Reiser DE, Schroder AK. *Patient Interviewing: The Human Dimension.* Baltimore, MD: Williams & Wilkins; 1980.
3. Rosen, DH. *Dr. Nada Live at the Tiny Tavern.* https://www.youtube.com/watch?v=0TUSNrU7f7A. Accessed November 15. 2016.
4. Lear MW. *Heartsounds.* New York: Pocket Books; 1981.
5. Engel G. A life setting conducive to illness: the giving-up/given-up complex. *Ann Intern Med.* 1968;679:293–300.
6. Schmale AH. Giving up as a final common pathway to changes in health. In: *Psychosocial Aspects of Physical Illness.* Vol. 8, Advances in Psychosomatic Medicine. Basel: Karger; 1972:20–40.

7. Moos RH, Tsu VD. Crisis of physical illness. In: Moos RH, ed. *Coping with Physical Illness*. New York: Plenum; 1977:3–21.
8. Kopacz DK. *Re-humanizing Medicine*. Washington, DC: Ayni Books; 2013.
9. Rosen DH. *Transforming Depression: Healing the Soul Through Creativity*. New York: Penguin Group; 1993.
10. Kleinman A, Eisenberg L, Good B. Culture, illness and care: clinical lessons from anthropologic and cross-cultural research. *Ann Intern Med*. 1975;88:251–258.

## SUGGESTED READINGS

Grooves JE. Taking care of the hateful patient. *N Engl J Med*. 1978;298:883–887.

Lipp MR. *Respectful Treatment: The Human Side of Medical Care*. Hagerstown, MD: Harper & Row; 1977.

# 7

# THE NATURE OF THE HEALING PROCESS

The main reason for healing is love.
—Paracelsus

## HEALING AND NATURAL SYSTEMS: THE DISTINCTION BETWEEN CURING AND HEALING

Every so often one hears about some "miraculous recovery" in medicine. A man with advanced metastatic cancer suddenly goes into remission and all traces of malignancy seem to have vanished, a woman terminal with a brain tumor defies the odds and continues to live, and so on. Often, such stories have the potential for sensationalism and are reported in the popular media for dramatic effect; at times, they are exaggerated. Yet, such "spontaneous" remissions, although rare, do occur. They have been described in the scientific literature and are not well understood. Furthermore, less extreme forms of psychological control over physical processes abound. We all know of the dying man who "made it" to his birthday, or of the mother who "held on" until she was reunited with her child. The fact that such phenomena have been regarded more from the perspective of sentiment than science should not discourage our curiosity and willingness to wonder about such things rationally and scientifically. Perhaps if we could stop applying such terms as *miraculous* and *astonishing* to natural phenomena involving healing (extreme and not so extreme), we would begin to understand them better. And really, we should not be so astonished. Healing is basic—a natural, integral aspect of all living systems. In truth, what should amaze us is only the extent to which this has been forgotten. As doctors, we too often tend to overestimate our power, to assume we always can and should act. Too quickly we reach for drugs, defibrillators, and Teflon grafts. Too frequently we forget that all such devices—no matter how wonderful in the right context—are only adjuncts to, or substitutes for, natural healing.

Healing is an intrinsic activity in all natural systems. Yet, perhaps this is not underscored enough by clinicians when discussing the role it plays in the recovery process. A dear friend of Uyen, whom we shall call Fran, gave the example of a computer software analyst who failed to troubleshoot a problem by going through the corrective processes, yet was able to resolve the issue simply by rebooting the entire system. Rebooting the system is analogous to our body's natural ability to heal without a prescriptive measure; akin to self-debugging. By design, the human body has an intrinsic ability to renew itself and heal (a property that does not get the attention it deserves when discussing a plan of care). Fran considered this IT analogy following a discussion we had on her distressing medical experience in which she was bounced around from her Ob-Gyn to several specialists for input on why she had urinary retention after an unremarkable, uncomplicated delivery in which she gave birth to a healthy baby. The illness experience required 6 months of self-catheterization, which left her shaken up. It seemed clear to Uyen, on hearing the story, that her friend's body simply healed on its own time, but the uncertainty and significance of this healing property was not communicated fully in terms of what she valued in recovery, except by 1 physician of 4 she had seen. Here is her story, in her own words:

> Having to endure the traumatic experience of losing basic biological functions of your body after giving birth was just that—traumatic and terrifying. The initial trauma was compounded by being bounced around from one specialist to another, all four of them not being able to provide any concrete cause for the problem, let alone a resolution or course of treatment to cure my issues. Added to this, I recognized that my medical issue may be a common, everyday occurrence to these specialists, but it wasn't to me, their patient. So treating me like I'm a statistic or just another case study was the final straw to my emotional turmoil. I was scared my life would never be normal again. It was only when my urologist finally sat down with me, empathized with my pain and fear, and provided some hope by sharing another patient's story and her similar prognosis that my anxiety was quelled. He did not provide me with a guarantee, but he listened and gave me advice that mattered to me: tips on what body signals to look for as indicators my condition was improving. He asked me to take action and stay the course with him by following up with him quarterly. That was all I could hope for and he gave me that.
>
> Bedside manners and empathy go a long way when medicine, treatment, and cures are not an option. Doctors often forget their profession is not only to resolve the medical problem at hand, but also it is to help their patient. Or is that too presumptive?

Fran was very emotional and aggrieved when sharing this experience, as if it had just happened. In hindsight, she recalled that all doctors said something to the effect of the uncertainty of her prognosis and, basically, that recovery (if so) was a waiting game. This was not couched in the framework of the body's natural healing properties. To be fair, Fran was not sure whether hearing this alone would have been enough, but what carried her through this trying period was her urologist's display of *acceptance* (listening. receiving, acknowledging her illness experience and its uncertainty), *empathy* (an understanding of her suffering diffused Fran's frustration and aided in recovery from the initial communication breakdown), *conceptualization* (self-awareness, sharing another patient's similar story to decrease anxiety and hold hope when uncertainty loomed, empowerment in identifying small changes in bodily function to gain some signpost for measuring progress), and *competency* (integrating foundational principles in managing her illness skillfully, recognizing the intrinsic property of healing, providing a timeline for future visits to return to her doctor for quarterly follow-ups).

Healing takes place at all levels of the systems hierarchy. Using a general systems approach, we know that every level or part influences that whole, and vice versa. Unless we have become completely numb, we also see the poetry inherent in this truth and stand in awe of the mysterious forces that spark life and promote healing. This is true whether it occurs on a subcellular level with replicating DNA, at the cellular level with billions of new cells replacing dead cells every day, or at the organ tissue level with the regeneration of vital functioning and wound healing. On a personal level, we know how important the human spirit and will to live are to a patient recovering from an illness. We are aware of the immensely healing properties of human relationships in their own right, whether they are the bond between mother and child, compassion toward a patient, or the love of a suffering person's family. Beyond this, we recognize that cultures, nations, societies, and the biosphere itself can promote healing by facilitating harmony, or can destroy it by fomenting fragmentation and chaos.

On a global scale, nuclear annihilation remains a significant and immediate threat (greater than the threat of climate change), admonishes Dr. Ira Helfand[1]—cofounder of Physicians for Social Responsibility and copresident of International Physicians for the Prevention of Nuclear War, which won the Nobel Peace Prize in 1985—during his presentation, "The Growing Danger of Nuclear War and What We Can Do About It." This is not simply political; it is compellingly sensible and, indeed, inevitable. Increasingly, physicians perceive their responsibility to protest this trend. The fate of the biosphere itself depends on nuclear restraint. Physicians who recognize this are acting logically on conclusions that a systems perspective forces all of us to reach.

To many, our injunction to this point may seem obvious. Still, the history of contemporary medicine and our current practices make it very clear we are not always doing what seems obvious. Far from it. Just look at our language, at the metaphors we so often choose. All too often we view ourselves as medical soldiers of a sort, waging war against disease. We speak of *combating* an infection. We *attack* the problem of heart disease. We try to *conquer* cancer. In short, medicine is a battle. It is war. Disease is an evil invader that has landed on the patients' shores from some remote and barbarous region. When patients begin to lose the battle against this invader, they call the doctor. Like a hired gunslinger or Samurai warrior, doctors take up the fray.

Of course, reality is very different. Illness always occurs in the *context* of a person's life. The settings in which illness emerges have much to do with a person's life: relationships, work, setbacks, triumphs, hopes, defeats, dreams, and struggles. Naturally, one should never be simplistic about this. It would be far too reductionistic to say, "He got cancer because he worried about his son" or "Her thyroid disease came about because her marriage was breaking up." It is equally foolish to deny all such connections and insist that illness is simply a random statistical event.

How such a narrowing perspective became so pervasive in medicine is complex. Regardless, the effects of this perspective have been troubling. What does such a perspective do, for example, to the doctor–patient relationship? The answer has to be: a great deal of harm. Viewing medicine as a battle all too often reduces patients to objects—a fragile boat, a rudderless frigate, a hapless barge of statistical misfortune tossed upon the stormy seas of illness. Doctors, in turn, view their responsibilities as a naval skirmish—a confrontation to be prepared for, fought, and won. Patients in this perspective are entirely passive. They hope only to be saved. Doctors send in their armada and try to occupy the disease's strategic islands; occasionally, doctors have to retreat. What they do not do is relate well to their patients. The families of patients are also relegated to the role of helpless bystander—worried figures huddling outside the hospital room, clutching hats and purses, waiting, hoping, praying for doctors to perform a miracle. With distressing regularity, families are excluded from any substantive involvement with physicians. All too often they are shunted aside, pushed into the corners of waiting rooms. There, they are expected to wait, drink tepid coffee from vending machines, peruse old magazines, and comply with the rules. They hover compliantly in the background while physicians, medicine's gladiators, unsheathe their swords and do battle with disease. Squandered are these powerful and potentially healing resources.

Beyond the damage all this does to patients and their families, all the opportunities of healing that are missed, what is just as troubling is the discouragement this promotes in physicians. Doctors, conceptualizing their efforts too exclusively in terms of absolute cure, have inadvertently relinquished critical roles, responsibilities, and opportunities that could bring considerable reward and meaning, which may be the saddest consequence of all. In our experience, young physicians who think solely in terms of cure risk terrible discouragement. It is *this* doctor people refer to when they speak of "burnout." Currently, there is an epidemic of such malaise among physicians. A 3-year study interval from 2011 to 2014 from a survey of 6880 physicians showed a statistically significant increase in burnout apparent in 24 medical specialties—an increase from 45% in 2011 to 54% in 2014—of physicians who reported at least 1 symptom of burnout.[2,3] Everywhere we hear of such burnout, "identity diffusion," and "job stress." Medicine *is* stressful; it always will be. But, some of the stress is actually the disheartenment that comes from misdirected energy, futile attempts to cure accompanied by an equally unfortunate failure to see the splendor and meaning in the healing work we really can do.

Doctors thus discouraged naturally try to compensate, but vacation homes, trips to Europe, 6-figure incomes, and fancy German automobiles do little to soften the core existential pain that results from a crisis of purpose and meaning. Medicine *is* a highly existential undertaking. As physicians, we confront life's greatest challenges—its highest joys, horrors, and mysteries. Above all, we confront mortality, our own as well as our patients'. This is truly a rare opportunity. It is also a stress. The practice of medicine is at the heart and soul of human realities that cannot be avoided, denied, or cast aside. As physicians, we *must* come to terms with life and death, and, although it is unquestionably a rare opportunity, young doctors need guidance and support if they are to master the pain and realize the opportunities. All too often, medical education has failed to meet this challenge.

Finally, even if we physicians ignore the existential core of what we are engaged in, our patients cannot. Patients today are clearly searching for something. Just look at the proliferation of self-help books, holistic health movements, natural products, diet-based therapies, mindfulness and meditation practices, naturopathy, acupuncture, homeopathy, and so on. According to the National Center for Complementary and Integrative Health's report, *The Use of Complementary and Alternative Medicine [CAM] in the United States*,[4] approximately 38% of adults and 12% of children use some form of CAM. Because of limited scientific data for most CAM therapies (not uncommon for such data to be misrepresented), patients are vulnerable to self-treat in a misguided way, but they are clearly seeking something. Instead of feeling smug, physicians should be asking: *What* are my patients seeking? Could the pursuit for unconventional therapies be a response to important, valid human needs? Could these be needs that contemporary medicine has ignored? Most of these newer movements emphasize the *human* needs of patients, including their spiritual and existential longings. We believe that until physicians take these matters seriously, people will continue to turn to those who do meet these needs, sometimes to healers with personal agendas, with adverse consequences to their health.

## THREE PATIENTS

In this section we discuss three patients who were trying to heal. In all three cases, opportunities were missed, not because people did not care, but because the physicians involved viewed their tasks too narrowly. With all these patients, we believe a healing partnership could have been possible had the doctors been able to see beyond the confines of a strictly biomedical perspective.

Some of you may notice something else. In all three cases, it was a medical student who first sensed something was wrong with the care each patient was receiving. Some will find this ironic, but no one should really be surprised. It is our hope medical students make a concerted effort to uphold the broad-minded, humanistic attitudes with which they entered this profession, well throughout training and into their clinical practice.

### Mrs. Dunbarton

Mrs. Dunbarton was a frail 82-year-old widow living in a pensioners' hotel near the Tenderloin District of San Francisco. A thin, wrenlike woman, she tended to wave her hands a great deal whenever she became excited, upset, or confused. At these times, her bony fingers would flutter like the wings of birds. The hand-waving occurred more often as she became increasingly forgetful and confused. She was also quite deaf. Despite these infirmities, however, she remained a pleasant, even-tempered woman, who always had a smile for people, including her nurses and doctors. In general, she greeted the world with compliance and trust, even when this was hardly warranted. Had she been wealthy, some con man no doubt would have taken advantage of her. In truth, she did not have a dime. Often, when Mrs. Dunbarton did not comprehend something, she would fake understanding. She would cock her head to one side, look up at the ceiling, and adopt a sage expression. At such moments, she appeared on the verge of saying something astonishing or profound, but the pronouncement never came. Instead, her mind just drifted off again.

Mrs. Dunbarton was in the hospital for the third time in 6 months, with pneumonia. The senior resident told Alice, the junior medical student taking care of Mrs. Dunbarton, that recurrences of pneumonia were not uncommon, but he also exhorted her to do a really good workup "just to be sure." This workup turned out to be both exhaustive and exhausting. They got more than enough sputum samples for culture and sensitivity analyses. There were radiographs of her chest, tomograms, and numerous skin tests for tuberculosis, coccidiomycosis, and histoplasmosis. Many tubes of blood were drawn. Mrs. Dunbarton was definitely getting a "million-dollar workup."

Ultimately, the investigation was negative. The radiographs showed the same degree of emphysema present as on the previous admissions. Her cardiac silhouette was small. Her EKG revealed low voltage but was otherwise normal. All cultures came back negative for any organism other than pneumococci. Thus, the medical team concluded confidently that this was, again, simply a case of pneumonia, and the team members left Mrs. Dunbarton's care to Alice, the medical student.

Quickly, the penicillin did its magic. Mrs. Dunbarton's fever came down. Her white count dropped once again below 10 000. Within a week, she was ready for discharge.

One morning, however, as Alice approached her bedside at a later hour than she ordinarily did, something caught her eye. Mrs. Dunbarton had a visitor. This was the first time Alice had ever seen Mrs. Dunbarton with anyone. Her visitor was a middle-aged black woman who exuded enthusiasm, vitality, and strength. When Alice approached the bedside, the visitor extended her hand and clasped Alice's firmly. She seemed eager to talk.

Mrs. Montgomery was her name. She was a volunteer from Mrs. Dunbarton's neighborhood church. During all three hospitalizations, Mrs. Montgomery had visited faithfully. For the first time, Alice learned the actual details of Mrs. Dunbarton's life outside the hospital. The old woman lived in poverty and squalor, spending her days in the lobby of a decaying downtown hotel where she and other pensioners rented small, peeling rooms. The tenants rarely went outside; there were too many muggings and everyone was in terror of venturing out of doors. During the winter, there were months without heat or hot water. Mrs. Montgomery tried as often as she could to visit her friend. On each trip she would bring Mrs. Dunbarton a boiled egg and a roll. Many Sundays she walked with her to church.

Learning of this stirred Alice deeply. She was shocked and unsettled by the stark reality of Mrs. Dunbarton's plight. That afternoon, Alice called the hospital social worker. It was the first time in Mrs. Dunbarton's three hospitalizations that Social Services had been contacted. A case worker was assigned who worked with Alice to inquire about obtaining additional Social Security benefits. They explored whether there might be a better place for Mrs. Dunbarton to live. Arrangements were made to have a daily hot meal brought to Mrs. Dunbarton by Meals on Wheels after her discharge.

Why had all of these remedies been so long in coming? After all, Mrs. Dunbarton had been a patient in a top-notch teaching hospital where the house staff worked hard and really cared. The problem lay not in anyone's intentions, but in the failure of her doctors to see beyond the organic part of her illness. Ironically, it had probably been the fact that Mrs. Dunbarton's disease was so *curable* that delayed and prevented proper comprehensive care. Pneumococcal pneumonia. It seemed so simple. An infection, an organism visualized, a drug to treat it, and a grateful patient who responded promptly. Unfortunately, until the third admission, her doctors—each time—returned Mrs.

Dunbarton to the same grim, depressing environment that may have contributed to compromising her resistance to developing pneumonia in the first place.

## Mrs. Vincent

Back in her teens, Bonnie Vincent looked forward to a promising future as a fashion model. Now, 10 years later, only traces of that halcyon time remain. On the mantle over the fireplace in her small, meticulously swept apartment there is a picture—a framed reproduction of a *Seventeen* magazine cover. Bonnie poses in the center, flanked by other lovely, long-legged, willowy girls with sparkling eyes and insouciant smiles. Seven ingénues have been posed together, winners of the magazine's beauty search. Bonnie is especially stunning—the tallest by several inches. Ten years later, Mrs. Vincent is 27, harder, perhaps wiser. The insouciance is gone. When people allude to that earlier time, she waves it away with a gesture of her hand and admonishes people, "All that was ages ago."

It *was* long ago. The present finds Mrs. Vincent thinner, wan, and visibly in pain. She is propped up in a hospital bed on three pillows. Yet, she is still very attractive and, if one looks closely, there are traces even now of a more innocent past. Her huge brown eyes are still strikingly beautiful, although they are now webbed with shadows and deep, furrowed lines. At 17, she was vibrant and slender; now, she is ashen and profoundly gaunt. She is dying.

Mrs. Vincent has an extremely malignant type of leukemia from which there is almost never a successful recovery. At this precise moment, however, and despite her deteriorating condition, she is trying to pack her overnight case. She is scheduled for discharge in 2 hours "Against Medical Advice." She still insists that she does not want to leave the hospital, but she silently accepts her fate. Her expression is cryptic. As she packs various items on her nightstand, she bites her lip, shrugs her shoulders, and perhaps reveals the faintest hint of a forming tear. There are no two ways about it; sick or not, dejected or not, the staff wants Mrs. Vincent out. She has definitely become *persona non grata* on ward 7-North.

To understand how this sorry state of affairs came about, one must go back 4 months to when Mrs. Vincent was first admitted to 7-North with the diagnosis of acute myeloid leukemia. At the time, she had been extremely ill with a high white blood cell count comprised almost exclusively of immature cells. She also had severe anemia. The residents treated her with transfusions of packed red cells, prednisone, IV antibiotics, and an aggressive course of chemotherapy. Mrs. Vincent responded quickly. The treatment also caused her considerable suffering. During chemotherapy, she lost nearly all of her hair and developed painful ulcerations in her mouth. It became almost impossible to swallow, and even attempting to eat was torture. She suffered severe shooting pains down her arms and legs, and she was racked by uncontrollable nausea and vomiting. Nevertheless, Mrs. Vincent cooperated with her treatment completely. She believed in the doctors who told her, "This will get you better."

Although she was always cooperative, from the outset Mrs. Vincent was not especially warm or open. She tended to be standoffish and exceedingly shy, responding to the staff's attempts at friendliness by pursing her lips, shrugging her shoulders, and looking away. At Mrs. Vincent's bedside, morning rounds would often go something like this:

RESIDENT: How are you feeling this morning?
MRS. VINCENT: (Purses lips, looks away, and shrugs.)
RESIDENT: We're going to be giving you another course of the vincristine today. Is that okay? Do you feel up to it?
MRS. VINCENT: (Purses lips, looks away, and shrugs; then, after a long pause, nods faintly.)

It was difficult to know whether her icy countenance reflected hostility, fear, or depression, but overall the residents found her to be a difficult patient to warm up to. They performed their duties conscientiously but without much sense of satisfaction or joy.

Mrs. Vincent had a frequent visitor—a burly, bearded black man in a peacoat who always wore dark sunglasses. He was completely unfriendly, and when he visited, everyone steered clear of them both. They argued often, quarrels that ended with the man storming out and Mrs. Vincent in tears. Mrs. Vincent also had two young daughters, 2 and 5 years old, but hospital policy prohibited their visiting. She kept pictures of them on her nightstand.

After the chemotherapy, Mrs. Vincent went into remission and was discharged. She declined follow-up in the outpatient clinic, stating she preferred to see her own doctor. As time passed, Mrs. Vincent was forgotten. Then, 4 months later, she was readmitted to 7-North, in severe relapse. Nobody was overjoyed. The rapidity and severity of her relapse spelled trouble. Everyone dreaded the next round of chemotherapy on this silent, emotionally inaccessible patient. Nevertheless, as duty required, they prepared to treat Mrs. Vincent once again. Only this time, they did not get very far.

"She's refusing chemotherapy," the intern told his senior resident. "She says she's willing to take the transfusions and antibiotics, but she doesn't want any more chemotherapy."

"We'll see about that," the resident replied. Now it was the resident's turn to strike out.

"She says she doesn't want to *leave* the hospital," the resident later told his attending, "but she refuses any more chemotherapy. She says if God wants to take her, then let God do his work."

"I'll talk with her about that," said the attending.

He did. Mrs. Vincent refused to budge. Negotiations continued for the next couple days without progress.

"I am prepared to die," the patient kept repeating.

Finally, house staff and attending all agreed. If Mrs. Vincent refused to accept appropriate medical treatment, they would discharge her, Against Medical Advice.

It was in this context that Joe, the medical student on the team, became concerned about his stoic patient's feelings and welfare. He asked us to visit Mrs. Vincent as part of a "Psychiatric Aspects of Medicine" course (see Rosen and Blackwell in "Suggested

Reading" at the end of the chapter). Joe had become alarmed when Mrs. Vincent refused a second course of chemotherapy, but even more alarmed when the medical team decided to begin forcing her to sign out Against Medical Advice. He feared that such a drastic measure would only compound her current suffering.

We talked with Mrs. Vincent at some length. Although she was not effusive, she was open and honest. We learned that, since the last hospitalization, she had separated from her husband, the sullen man in the peacoat. She said she was fed up with his infidelity, alcoholic excesses, and abusiveness toward her and the children. Yet regarding her current situation, she was adamant.

"No," she said to us, "No more chemotherapy. Absolutely not."

She wanted the doctors to treat her as best as they could. To make her comfortable, but not if that meant she would have to endure the "living hell" of chemotherapy again. She wanted to live, but added, "I'm not afraid to die."

Toward the end of our discussion, Mrs. Vincent revealed a cherished personal goal. She wanted to live long enough—just about 3 weeks—to complete divorce proceedings. This would ensure her daughters were safely in the custody of her mother, legally protected from the abusive father.

With tears flooding her eyes, she said, "This is really all I want. I'm not afraid of death," she said again.

She told us she was greatly comforted by her religious beliefs. Indeed, she had a theory about her own passing: God wanted children and beautiful young people in heaven too, so that it would not be filled with people who were old and debilitated.

With our support, Joe presented his findings to the rest of the team. He was inclined to think that Mrs. Vincent was depressed. He urged the house staff and attending physician to give him more time to form an alliance with the patient. Then, perhaps, he could convince Mrs. Vincent to be rational about accepting chemotherapy. During this discussion, the idea was never seriously considered that Mrs. Vincent might have a right to refuse the treatment.

The medical team agreed to an extension, but 2 days later Mrs. Vincent still had not budged. She had several more affable conversations with Joe in the interim and expressed increasing confidence that her life had not been in vain. But, on the matter of chemotherapy, she never wavered. Soon, Mrs. Vincent was discharged. Against Medical Advice. She died 2 weeks later in another hospital, dejected, with her divorce not yet final.

This clinical vignette raises many critical questions. Why did the healthcare system not at least attempt to respect her stated wishes and support the desires she cherished? Why was she not sent home, not with the hand-washing formula Against Medical Advice, but with essential medical advice, buoying support, and compassionate follow-up care by home visiting nurses and physicians? In a real sense, Mrs. Vincent was mistreated not because she had given up on life, but because she refused standard treatment—a treatment that, ironically, offered not a trace of a chance for a cure. She had stepped out of the established "system" and, as punitive as it may seem, she was left feeling abandoned with unnecessary suffering. Joe attempted to recognize her all-too-human yearnings. Unfortunately, as commonly happens, the medical team found a multitude of reasons to ignore him.

Why did this happen? Perhaps the medical staff members were so caught up in their own definition of curing disease that they lost sight of Mrs. Vincent herself, of her real desires at the close of her life, her own goals and needs. But, simply to condemn the doctors who cared for her is too easy and it does not help. Rather, we must try to empathize. This may provide some clues of why this tragedy happened. Often when there is no cure, doctors feel impotent and helpless—as if they have failed personally. This is irrational, of course, but terribly common. Far too often, doctors pressure themselves to achieve the impossible. They demand of themselves cures that simply do not exist and, in the process, forget that even when a cure is not possible, there still remain many opportunities to facilitate a healing process. Acceptance. Listening. Support. Keeping hope alive. Truly knowing what it means to walk in the patient's shoes and being able to communicate that knowledge. These are human acts, always available to physicians; interventions they can and sometimes must choose to make, especially when the hope for cure is long since past, when, as was true for Mrs. Vincent, the patient seeks not biomedical recovery, but compassionate, human support; spiritual transformation; and final peace—the healing people seek when they know death is at hand.

## Mr. Moore

First our pleasures die—and then
Our hopes, and then our fears—and when
These are dead, the debt is due,
Dust claims dust—and we die, too.

—Shelley

Picture an abandoned farmhouse. It is rotting somewhere out on a prairie where roads no longer go. Slowly, the skeleton of a place that once held life is baking to death in the harsh summer sun. Perhaps this is transpiring on some parched, waterless, indifferent Texas plain. The windows are shattered and long since devoid of any remaining glass. The rooms of the farmhouse are completely gutted and have been for years. A door still hangs by one rusty hinge. Now and again it flaps idly against its frame, stirred by some ghostly, invisible breeze.

Now, try to imagine the incredible physical deterioration that has taken place during the past 6 months in Mr. Alan Moore. He is 6 feet 3 inches but weighs only 107 pounds. Daily, he scorches with a body temperature of 101°F or more. Antipyretics and antibiotics fail repeatedly to bring his temperature down. Malignant melanoma has gutted and ravaged him. He is very close to the end of his life. Everywhere, throughout his body, tumor cells proliferate in uncontrolled anaplasty, choking out normal cells the way weeds crowd out healthy vegetation. His liver, bowel, and lungs are all terminally infested with histopathological chaos. Mr. Moore is 33 but he looks 50. Dissipation funnels through him like some hot Texas wind, and death peeks out surreptitiously from the shadows of his eyes, like a tramp hiding in the barn, waiting only for nightfall to make his final move. Mr. Moore never complains or makes demands, but from the hallway outside his room, one hears retching and choking, muted moans. Against the stark hospital wall one sees his emaciated shadow, like some ghostly Giaccometti sculpture, hunched over an emesis basin, throwing up incessantly. The end is proving to be horrible; there is just no way to soften or romanticize it.

We met Mr. Moore because his suffering affected one of our junior medical students very deeply. Paul had gone, as always, on daily rounds with his medical team. The junior resident was presenting the latest laboratory data, all of which confirmed Mr. Moore's relentless decline.

The group spoke well outside the patient's earshot. Finally, one of the residents, after crisply reciting the latest numbers, put Mr. Moore's chart back in the rack with a sigh. He then shrugged his shoulders, turned his palms upward toward the ceiling, and exclaimed, "Why isn't this patient dead?!"

He did not make this comment with any malice, but the next thing that happened was dramatic indeed.

Slowly, an intern on the case began to giggle. The attending put his fingers to his lips and tried, but failed, to suppress his own laughter. Soon, the whole thing broke wide open. Six doctors of varying age, rank, sex, and experience were all laughing, repeating over and over, "Why isn't this man dead?" Each time the question was repeated, the group would once again shake with laughter.

Doubtless, some would say that such behavior is scandalous, but we believe it is understandable. Human. The medical team, in our opinion, was releasing torrents of almost unbearable pain. The tears we saw streaming down their cheeks were not just tears of laughter. Practicing medicine can be very difficult.

Still, the question disturbed Paul. He presented Mr. Moore's case to us. Quite somber now, Paul again asked, "Why isn't this man dead?"

It was a good question. An important one.

Why indeed?

The first thing we asked Paul was if the medical team had shared its amazement with Mr. Moore. Had anyone asked *him* where he got the courage and strength to endure? Such a question, from our perspective, was not simply an admiring compliment. We *did* admire Mr. Moore; but, as physicians, we knew it was more important to understand him. Consider the parallel: Almost any doctor would feel comfortable asking her patient with arthritis how, despite advanced debility, she still managed to sew and do the dishes. Was asking Mr. Moore how he endured his disfigurement and pain any different? Yet, because of the inhibitions and taboos that people feel about death, no one asked. Thus, Paul's reply was not unexpected.

"No," he said, "We routinely discuss his case in the hallway, outside of his room. We only spend brief moments . . . actually with him."

Paul continued, "When we are with him, it's mostly to monitor his drugs, like his pain medications. You know, whether he needs more or less. That kind of thing. We always tell him to let us know if he needs more. Nobody wants the poor guy to suffer. But, you know, we don't get into what's really going on with the guy."

"Let's go in and see him."

Paul nodded solemnly and loosened the knot in his tie.

When we entered the patient's darkened room, we entered a cathedral of silence, a silence broken only by the rustle of bed sheets and a low continuous murmur of pain. Mr. Moore was extremely cachectic. He resembled a survivor of Nazi atrocities. But as hideous as his physical condition was, his expression was lively and alert. We had hardly expected this! To our considerable surprise, his eyes were bright, engaging, and (dare we say?) full of hope. He was in obvious pain. Shortly after we entered the room, he suddenly clutched his abdomen, gasped, and began to retch and heave. He groped feebly for his emesis basin, apologizing meekly, and slumped over it, commencing to vomit.

One of us put her hand on his shoulder. Another held the emesis basin under his chin. We tried our best to comfort him. Finally, Mr. Moore again grew quiet. The paroxysm appeared to pass. We introduced ourselves. Was he comfortable enough to be interviewed?

"Oh yes! Sure!"

In a raspy voice he said he had been looking forward to the interview and was feeling "all right."

It was obviously a painful, faltering start. However, once the interview had gotten under way, everyone became quite engrossed, including Mr. Moore.

One of us finally popped the question, "How do you keep going? ... It's so *severe*. Your illness ... the way you keep going—it's remarkable."

Mr. Moore smiled.

"Maybe I'm stubborn. All I know is, I'm not ready to die. Nuh uh! Not yet!"

During the course of the interview, Mr. Moore became increasingly energetic. Especially, his eyes sparkled as he talked lovingly of his wife. He told us also about his parents. It gave him great pleasure that, in recent years, he had once again grown close to them. "It's amazing how much they've matured in the last few years!" he laughed. He and his wife were planning to spend the summer with them. They had a cottage on Lake Huron. It would be the perfect place to recuperate, draw, and paint.

Drawing and painting—these were things he had done much earlier in his life but had somehow grown to neglect in recent years. He had always seemed too busy, too caught up in one thing or another to find the time. Now, just recently, he had reembraced his old love. Once again, he found himself seized by an insatiable passion to create.

"Art is one of the things I have to live for," he said. "Does that make any sense?"

Several of us nodded.

We discovered he had been drawing and painting almost nonstop since his most recent admission to the hospital. Some of his drawings were "visualizations." These he had done in conjunction with his irradiation and chemotherapy. Although his physicians had been skeptical, saying only, "Do whatever you want," Mr. Moore believed these exercises might be helpful. He worked with a psychologist interested in such matters. Collaborating, they mapped out a strategy whereby he would draw pictures to aid his own immune system. Many of his drawings depicted his image of his own white blood cells fighting the cancer. He portrayed them as powerful, ravenous warriors, unstoppable in their appetites, gnawing away relentlessly and finally overpowering the ugly, ill-formed cancer cells.

Suddenly, his face lit up. "Would you like to see some of my work?"

A rustle in the room. A shifting of feet. Then, nods and smiles.

Characteristic of his independence and strong will, Mr. Moore insisted on getting out of bed unassisted. Very painfully and very slowly he hobbled over to his dresser and opened the top drawer where he kept his drawing tablet. Cradling it in his arms, he inched his way back to the hospital bed. But now, back in bed with his artist's notebook open, animation and vigor seemed to return. Enthusiastically, he began showing us his drawings, describing them, relishing them. The first was a portrait of a woman he had done before entering the hospital. It was executed in charcoal—large gashing strokes, jagged intersecting black lines, bold and incomplete. Starkly, in black and white, the portrait conveyed to us the artist's angst: rage, despair, fury, and loneliness, all these feelings at once.

He showed us this piece hastily and without comment.

"Here's another one," he said, flipping the page. "I think you'll like this one."

Now he showed us a colorful pastel. This drawing had been completed more recently, shortly after he was admitted to the hospital. It depicted how the radiation treatment (drawn as multicolor "rainbow energy") maimed and killed the cancer cells while his white blood cells victoriously gobbled up the injured and dead cancer cells.

"Now," he said with unmistakable pride, "Here's my favorite!"

He showed us a drawing done the day before. It was another portrait, again of a woman. But, unlike the first one, this piece was full of softness and tender, beautiful detail. He had executed it with very fine, delicate strokes. He had filled the page completely with shading and color. The portrait was so realistic it seemed almost like a photograph.

Paul, the medical student, exclaimed with delight, "That's your wife, isn't it? Wow! It looks just like her."

Mr. Moore turned to Paul and grinned. "Yes, it is. It is my wife. Do you like it? I did this one with a whole lot of love in my heart! It shows, huh?"

"Wow!" Paul said, drawing closer, "I mean *that's* really something!" Without thinking about it, Paul now reached out his hand and touched Mr. Moore. With the index finger of his left hand, he very delicately traced the drawing. With his right hand, he now clasped his patient's shoulder.

"You like it?" Mr. Moore asked, looking up at Paul, visibly beaming.

"Yeah!" Paul replied, "Oh, yeah! Oh, yeah! Really!"

Several years have passed since that day, when we all talked with Mr. Moore. We still muse from time to time and wonder: Might he still be alive? It is unlikely. Of course, if we really wanted to find out, we could. Perhaps we prefer to remember Mr. Moore just as we last saw him, with Paul's hand on his shoulder, his eyes full of excitement, joy, and pride.

Who can assess the true worth of a human being's effort to communicate the meaning of life, even as he is leaving it? Our meeting with Mr. Moore was remarkably meaningful for us all. As human beings, we were touched. As physicians, a number of things struck us as quite remarkable. During the interview, Mr. Moore never once grimaced with pain. He showed no sign of feeling nauseated. He did not once vomit or retch. When he showed us his artwork, he especially appeared to be utterly pain-free.

Why?

Equally noteworthy was the lack of awareness among Mr. Moore's physicians that he drew and painted at all.

Why?

The residents knew vaguely about his "visualizations." Because he had insisted on being allowed to try to do the visualizations, they had even given their begrudging permission, but they acted as though such endeavors were trivial and slightly far out.

Why?

Scientific evidence supporting the effectiveness of visualizations (more aptly known as guided visual imagery today) was limited when Mr. Moore's case was initially presented. It has grown over the years, although perhaps not on the radar of many still. To Mr. Moore, this therapy clearly meant a great deal. Why was this trivialized and ignored? In addition, Mr. Moore was a member of an Eastern religious sect. Part of his worship included daily prayer and meditation, yet none of this was deemed at all important by the medical staff.

Why?

Still other questions arise: Does the will to live help one to go on in the face of death? This notion has long been entertained anecdotally. Is it true? If so, how does it work? Has it been studied enough? Or at all?

Do creative pursuits, such as Mr. Moore's drawing and painting, conceivably decrease the experience of pain? How does this happen? Does being creative somehow promote healing? If so, how does this function at the level of brain chemistry? Do the intangibles of hope, love, faith, and belief reinforce a person's will to live? What is the effect of loving? Of being loved? How did Mr. Moore's deep love for his wife affect him? His rapprochement with his parents?

What of prayer, meditation, faith, and belief in God? Over and over our patients tell us these things are very important. There is a growing body of research in these areas that is beyond the scope of this text. How has such a fertile field of investigation gone uncultivated and allowed to lie fallow under our scientific noses for so long?

## Touching

Those of you who are observant may have noted that a significant part of Mr. Moore's interaction with us involved touching. At the start of the interview, there was little physical contact. Indeed, the first thing that greeted the students had been a sepulchral somberness, a room filled with so much that was sad, ominous, and dark—a room that resonated with the sound of human pain. By the end of the interview, however, everyone had drawn closer. Paul and Mr. Moore were touching each other. The other students kept reaching out. This was no social contrivance or cookbook recipe regarding "physical contact in the medical interview." Far from it. What happened between Mr. Moore and the students was both natural and extremely powerful—a consequence of their growing rapport, deepening empathy, and budding awareness of a mutually shared humanness. This closeness was all the more powerful because it grew like a bright flower in the shadow of life's ultimate darkness: death. Perhaps the most important message of all that Mr. Moore and the students conveyed to each other came not in words at all, but in physical contact, in the touch of a hand. Listen to Lewis Thomas (in *The Youngest Science*) on the matter[5]:

> Medicine was once the most respected of all the professions. Today, when it possesses an array of technologies for treating (or curing) disease which were simply beyond comprehension a few years ago, medicine is under attack for all sorts of reasons. Doctors, the critics say, are applied scientists, concerned only with the disease at hand, but never with the patient as an individual, whole person. They do not really listen. They are unwilling or incapable of explaining things to sick people or their families. They make mistakes in their risky technologies; hence the rapidly escalating cost of malpractice insurance. They are accessible only in their offices in huge, alarming clinics or within the walls of terrifying hospitals. The word "dehumanizing" is used as an epithet for the way they are trained and for the way they practice. The old art of medicine has been lost, forgotten . . . . (ref. 5, pp. 55–60)

What is it that people have always expected from doctors? How, indeed, has the profession of medicine survived for so much of human history? Doctors as a class have always been criticized for their deficiencies. Montaigne in his time, Moliere in his, and Shaw had less regard for doctors and their medicine than today's critics. What on earth were the patients of physicians in the 19th century and the centuries before, all the way back to professional ancestors, the shamans of prehistory, hoping for when they called for a doctor? In the years of the great plagues, when carts came through the town streets each night to pick up the dead and carry them off for burial, what was the function of the doctor? Bubonic plague, typhus, tuberculosis, and syphilis were representative examples of a great number of rapidly progressive and usually lethal infections, killing off most of the victims no matter what was done by the doctor. What did doctors do, when called out at night to visit the sick for whom they had nothing to offer for palliation, much less cure?

Well, one thing they did, early in history, was plainly magic. Shamans learned their profession the hardest way; they were compelled to go through something like a version of death itself, personally, and when they emerged, they were considered qualified to deal with patients. They had epileptic fits, saw visions and heard voices, lost themselves in the wilderness for weeks on end, fell into long stretches of coma, and, when they came back to life, they were licensed to practice, dancing around the bedside, making smoke, chanting incomprehensibilities, and *touching* the patient everywhere. The touching was the real professional secret—never acknowledged as the central, essential skill—always obscured by the dancing and the chanting, but always busily there, the laying on of hands.

There, we think, is the oldest and most effective act of doctors: the touching. Some people don't like being handled by others, but not, or almost never, sick people. They *need* to be touched, and part of the dismay in being very sick is the lack of close human contact. Ordinary people, even close friends, even family members, tend to stay away from the very sick, touching them as infrequently as possible for fear of interfering or catching the illness or just fear of bad luck. Doctors' oldest skill in the trade was to place their hands on the patient.

Pause and consider for a moment the real significance of touch, the craving that human beings have to be embraced when they are suffering and in pain. When we cease to romanticize the phenomenon and consider it objectively, our amazement hardly diminishes. In fact, it is bound to grow. As documented by James Lynch,[6] there is astounding power in a human's touch. Yet touch appears to be on the decline in medicine, too often denigrated, ignored, and unappreciated.

The sheer complexity of modern medicine—its growing anonymity—discourages expressions of connectedness, closeness, and warmth. As Thomas[5] observes, in our modern medical complexes, the most protracted personal interaction a patient often has occurs not with a doctor or a nurse, but with a clerk at the admissions desk. The most intimate aspects of a person's life elude the doctor but are fed, instead, into an accountant's computer terminal, to be spit out onto an insurance form.

"Name?"

"Address?"

"Mother's maiden name?"

"Relative to contact?"

Each question is answered dutifully, as though by rote. During the process, the interrogator seldom nods or even makes eye contact.

"Annual income?"

"Place of employment?"

The patient replies obediently. The computer's keyboard clatters. Hieroglyphics of a life appear on a screen.

Touch, intimacy, closeness, a sense of belonging—many fear their disappearance from medicine hurts patients deeply. Sadly, this is true, but we worry about something beyond this. Such alienation is also taking its toll on doctors.

One of the great joys of medicine comes from the fact that the work we do is often highly meaningful. We should never forget how truly blessed we are to have a profession, so full of purpose, importance, and meaning. A six-figure income pales in comparison with this kind of wealth. Often, however, our work is also draining emotionally and spiritually. Sometimes we must endure a kind of pain and responsibility that are truly excruciating and harrowing. The essence of what we do is connected to what is most elemental and mysterious in life. Above all, we confront life's deepest riddle: death. We cannot and should not flee this. The evasion just will not succeed. Physicians must come to grips with their philosophical burdens and opportunities. It goes with the territory, as they say; there really is no choice. To flee from these things only leads to numbness, loss of purpose, confusion, and professional misery. The task of educators is not to find shortcuts to escape hatches; it is to help students master what they face, increase their wisdom, and grow from the challenges they confront. This is true whether the challenge is a new procedure to be learned or the human dimension of a physician–patient encounter. Much of what we fear, and long for, is embodied in the doctor–patient relationship and that most elemental part of it: the human touch.

Reaching out. Healing. It can be beautiful, but it can also be terrifying, exposing us to some of the most painful and trying of human situations. We should not make light of it or blame any lapses simplistically on "technologies." The pain of dying is hard, very hard. This was true long before CAT scans, comprehensive metabolic panels, and protein electrophoresis. The loneliness of illness, the sheer awfulness of dying are profound. These things frighten us to the core and always have. How naive to blame all our dread on a fickle and faddish infatuation with high technology. Let us be honest; it is frightening to be a doctor. It always has been. Yet, if doctors can reach out, can touch, can reach across that dreadful existential chasm, so much that is profound, inspiring, beautiful, and uplifting really can be achieved. The doctor–patient relationship *is* astounding and incredibly beautiful, but we should stop pretending it is easy. Sometimes, touching *can* help, amazingly so. Take Mr. Moore. Suddenly, he is no longer an apparition; he is again a human being, a person with hopes *even when he is in excruciating pain*. He is someone alive and sentient with very simple yet vital human needs. Above all, he is a person who needs others, someone longing for human contact. Like his ancestors through the centuries, he is afraid and longs for human touch. Responding to this need is one of doctors' most ancient and critical responsibilities. When we touch Mr. Moore, we are not simply being supportive of our patient. We are engaged in healing, responding to his anguish. It is all part of our calling, one of the demands we must be prepared to make of ourselves.

One final point about touching: It is connected closely with what we refer to in Chapter 1 as *acceptance*, a basic principle of medicine as a human experience. Think about it. We begin life as physical organisms. Long before language and abstraction develop, we know the world through our sensations, through what we feel. It is through touch that we begin to identify love, safety, and, indeed, survival.

Mother holds baby. Baby touches mother. It *is* a lovely picture. We could say the sight is *touching*. This is also the biology of survival. Human touch is one of the first and most highly critical events in the process of mother–infant bonding.

Currently, our scientific model tends to regard such matters as trivial. In general, we have failed to recognize the rich vein of important knowledge that awaits a curious investigator. it is more than a vein; it is a mother lode. As Lynch[6] has shown, a scientific inquiry into the impact on patients of touching tells us so much of critical importance. However, such matters are apt to be ignored until medicine begins to grasp their significance within the systems perspective. Until then, all these matters will remain enshrouded in folklore and sentiment—or worse still, be belittled as "unscientific." For the most part, they await the inquiry of perspicacious and curious minds.

## HEALING AND THE BIOPSYCHOSOCIAL MODEL

Currently, medicine is a house divided. We are cleaved painfully on many issues: private practice versus publicly funded medicine, specialists versus generalists, physicians providing healthcare versus nonphysicians providing healthcare. The list goes on and on. At times, the only thing that does seem to unite us is our shared belief that something is wrong with medicine, perhaps desperately wrong. We live in the wealthiest nation in the world and find ourselves devoting ever greater proportions of our total budget to healthcare. With each passing year, people seem more unhappy, more alienated, and more angry at American medicine. On the other side, exasperated physicians respond defensively and ask bitterly, "What do people want anyway?" Anger, disappointment, and pain; these emotions, more than any sense of common resolve, seem to be what unite us. As a consequence, many of us find ourselves longing for the "good old days." Then, we like to fantasize, everything was harmonious, happy, and whole.

Of course, the good old days never really existed. People were no more trusting of physicians in Montaigne's time than they are today. Leaving aside our current deficiencies and excesses as a profession, ambivalence about doctors is probably inevitable. In truth, it is inconceivable that a calling linked so closely to life and death, to human fate, would ever be regarded without profound conflict. Despite the currently politicized climate and a nimble rhetoric of holism, the problems that beset us are not new, and the solutions certainly no simpler. If only they were simple! For anyone who does not succumb to easy answers, the current climate is disquieting.

Increasingly, the schisms that divide us seem to grow: "holistic" versus "technological," "primary care" versus "specialty care," the "art" of medicine versus the "science" of medicine. Whatever dichotomy one selects, there is clearly a *perceived* schism between "scientific" medicine and "humanistic" medicine. It is the sort of nonsense that would not be so serious if it did not threaten patients. Permit us to concretize this. Consider once again the medical management of Mr. Moore. Recall that with begrudging "permission" from his medical team Mr. Moore undertook some visualization exercises. Here, indeed, is a case in point. The time will come when, through science, the efficacy of visualizations will have been proved or disproved. Let us presume for a moment that the outcome is positive. Hopefully, although by no means automatically, such proof can lead to acceptance and application of such techniques by "traditional" medicine. Until then, most reasonable people would agree there is little apparent *harm* in visualizations. This is especially true if patients believe in them and embrace them as part of their treatment, in concert with established forms of therapy. Clearly, Mr. Moore was no fanatic; along with his visualizations, he accepted and had faith in the chemotherapy and radiation treatments his physicians provided. Mr. Moore's care thus seems to have been logical, uncontroversial. Yet, considerable controversy actually coalesces around even so seemingly simple and rational a care plan as this. Especially, feelings and rhetoric run high on both sides over the issue of "scientific" versus "naturalistic" medicine.

Let us elaborate on this controversy and begin by articulating, as best we can, the views of both camps in this controversy. On one side, we have the views of what we shall call, for simplicity's sake, the "holistic" movement in medicine. Proponents on this side of the schism argue that biotechnical medicine must pay attention to the importance of self-healing, which the modern medical establishment perhaps ignores. So far, so good. Who could disagree? However, from here the rhetoric may expand, becoming more strident and extreme. Some say: Not only should Mr. Moore engage in visualizations, he should eschew the harmful drugs and chemicals that establishment doctors are forcing on him. All such substances are part of a medical conspiracy, worse than poison. He should turn to nature for healing. No more drugs, no more synthetic vitamins. Only *natural* will do. Honey, please; no sugar. From here, Mr. Moore may be exhorted to meditate, to think about the unity of nature and all of life. He may be exhorted to adopt a macrobiotic diet and renounce the evils of Western scientific thought.

What about the other side of the schism? The traditional Western medical establishment? Is this camp really any more reasonable? Here, too, the reasoning probably starts out sensibly. *Of course,* some doctors assert, patients *should* be allowed to have a say in their own treatment. "Obviously" the patient's wishes and religious beliefs should be considered. Still, as the passions behind the argument swell, you hear the prejudices churning underneath that rational surface. As for people who believe in meditation, diet, and prayer—well, these people are at best well-intentioned and at worst off the grid. Many physicians try to adopt a stance of reasonableness in the face of alternative therapies, but underneath they are quite incensed and, if prodded, explore, telling you the entire holistic health movement is really a lot of nonsense.

Obviously taken to extremes, neither camp is "right." There is truth on both sides of the chasm. How, then, has it happened that each side regards the other as so incorrigible and willful? At the core, what is wrong actually has nothing to do with intentions or intelligence. There are bright and sincere people polemicizing on both sides of the schism. What we are actually witnessing is confusion, a confusion that results inevitably from an inadequate underlying scientific model. Despite obvious differences in the scientific model that each side invokes, in critical respects they are surprisingly similar. Especially, both camp use models that rely heavily on cause and effect, and reductionism. This is a provocative assertion. Allow us to expand: The antimedical "holistic" camp invokes a model of nature that is essentially identical to that found in all prescientific cultures (of which it is an example). Such cultures attempt to explain natural events by "displacing upward" on the systems hierarchy. For example, these cultures explain illness by invoking causes that are larger, greater, and more removed than people themselves. Thus the ancients blamed illness on "the gods" or malalignment of the stars.

Although the direction of displacement in this model is upward, its effect is no less reductionistic. Nor is this "displacement upward" restricted to primitive cultures and historical antiquity. Some forms of contemporary psychological reductionism, for example, are similar and just as unhelpful. Thus, some people assert naively that a person got an ulcer "because he is unconsciously mad," or a woman developed asthma because she "could not tolerate separation from her mother." Here, the displacement is upward from the ailing body to the mysterious unconscious with its unseen gods and demons. Likewise, displacement upward is the favored etiological explanation for the current "naturalistic" movements within medicine. For instance, so-called "iridologists" claim they can discern all diseases by looking into the eye—a sort of window to the body and soul. The counterpart in primitive cultures would be witch doctors who discern patterns in the rocks and bones they scattered on the ground. The problem in many diseases is purported by these "naturalistic" practitioners to be some imbalance, a disruption in the harmony of yin and yang, which in turn reflects discordance contrary to some higher universal balance. Such thinking, of course, is no different from the ancients who cited horoscopes and pointed to the confluence or divergence of certain stars.

Western "scientific" medicine, with its emphasis on objective evidence and Cartesian dualism, as well as reductionistic explanations of cause and effect, is far more rational empirically, but it is equally hobbled ultimately by its insistence on a *linear quid pro quo* to explain all natural phenomena. It seeks etiological explanations by *displacing downward*. To explain illness at the person level, biomedicine attempts to *analyze* the problem (which means to break things into smaller component parts), and hopes in this way to find the "ultimate truth" at a cellular, molecular, atomic, or subatomic level. The biomedical model inherently encourages physicians to confuse "smaller" with "closer to the truth."

Throughout this book we have advocated the biopsychosocial model, based on systems theory, as a sensible and practical path toward reconciling many apparent polarities and schisms. We believe that proponents of the holistic movement in healthcare cannot be entirely ignorant and without substance. They are resonating with some legitimate perception on the part of many people, not all of whom are ignorant. At the same time, many scientifically committed physicians, including us, are dismayed by the complete noblesse oblige and uncomprehending caprice with which such movements commingle common sense, conjecture, and quackery. We acknowledge that physicians are not always effective at protecting patients from the dangers of their own biomedical excesses and too often ignore natural, intrinsic modes of healing. Thus, it comes as no surprise that many "naturalistically" inclined people view physicians with fear. Physicians are also accused by this movement, correctly, of failing often to see the suffering person who exists behind the radiographs and enzymes profiles. We physicians seem so eager to isolate (at considerable cost) and analyze smaller and smaller parts of the human whole. This can be wrong, but a rejection of the scientific method would be equally destructive and absurd. As we stated at the outset, solutions are not simple. However, at the very least, the biopsychosocial model shows how many apparently disparate "truths" are actually equally valid phenomena observed *at different levels* of the systems hierarchy. This model points a way toward a view of people as not *either* heart-and-soul *or* cells-and-mitochondria but *both—all of this* and much, much more—functioning as a fantastic whole of incredible intricacy, coherency, purpose, and design.

## MEDICINE'S EXISTENTIAL QUEST

In Andre Malraux's famous novel, *Man's Fate*,[7] there is a depiction of altruism in the face of death. The novel concerns the struggle of Communist freedom fighters in China during the revolution. The scene takes place in 1927. The protagonist is Katow, a hardened Russian revolutionary now fighting with the Chinese Communists. Katow is no stranger to death; he fought in the Russian Revolution, was shot at by a firing squad, and was a prisoner of hard labor. Now, he is a prisoner again, among many, all of whom are condemned to die. The less prominent and influential will be put to death by shooting before a firing squad. Important and influential people, such as Katow and his friend Keo, are to be cremated alive in the boiler of a locomotive. From outside the prison, the condemned hear the piercing wail of the locomotive's whistle. Each peal signals that another prisoner is being burned to death. Both Katow and Keo possess a cyanide tablet. Now, groping in the dark, Katow discerns that Keo is dead. He has already swallowed his poison. In the darkness, Katow hears two young boys, revolutionaries but barely out of their teens, sobbing in terror. He makes one of the most difficult decisions of his life; breaking the tablet in half, he gives each of them one-half tablet of his cyanide.

It is winter 1981 in Washington, DC. In a horrifying airline disaster, a commercial jetliner, its wings heavily iced, has skidded off the end of the runway and plunged into the Potomac. Hundreds die. Commuter traffic stops as horrified onlookers behold the catastrophe in stunned silence from an overhead bridge. Suddenly, a Washington office worker who was commuting home emerges from his car, proceeds to the riverbank, and leaps head first into the water. Nearly losing his own life in the process, he is able to pluck a drowning passenger from certain death.

In Canada, an athletic young man develops an osteosarcoma. In rapid succession he experiences amputation, chemotherapy, and radiation treatment. Equally important, he now must adjust to a severely altered self-image. He is suddenly "an invalid," a "cancer sufferer," and "disabled." His name is Terry Fox. In a stupendous feat that combines obstinacy with courage and ecstasy with suffering, Fox attempts to run across the continent to raise money for cancer research. As most people know, he did not make it. He died 2000 miles into his odyssey after metastases developed in his lungs. By the time of his death, however, he had galvanized the pride of an entire nation, inspired countless young people with cancer, and generated a huge outpouring of financial support for cancer research and treatment. His was truly an inspired act of creative madness; it made no sense and yet it made so *much* sense. It was the sort of divine folly that only human beings seem to be driven to and capable of.

These vignettes are especially dramatic, inspiring instances of human transcendence. Through heroes such as these we all hold up a mirror to ourselves and feel heartened. They remind us of the beauty, courage, and grace of which people are capable. (We already have far too many reminders of our baseness, destructiveness, pursuit of power, and arsenals of death.) Ultimately, heroes would be less important than they are, however, if they did not also help us to hold up smaller mirrors to our quieter, more personal moments of courage, love, creativity, and hope: A volunteer who will never make the newspapers reads passages of great literature every Thursday to a woman who is blind. A young man with Ivy League credentials and a promising job in a law firm joins the Peace Corps. A busy resident physician in pediatrics is about to rush by the room of a frightened 10-year-old. She has much to do—IVs to start, physicals to be performed, medication orders to be written—but something makes her stop. She enters and, for a few minutes, plays with the child, tucks him into bed, and kisses him goodnight. Her kindness will never be reported. In fact, she herself regards it as far too trivial to mention the next day on morning rounds. Yet, indelibly, undeniably, in the mind of the child, it has occurred. It may be that the most profound evidence of our humanness is not to be found in instances of great heroism, but in small, everyday acts—the touch of a hand, a look of understanding, a willingness to really listen. Reflect on the medical students' actions with the three patients in this chapter and on the vignettes presented throughout this book. It is heartening to remember that our profession has the real possibility of remaining a healing profession, and it is encouraging beyond measure that our students are so often at the vanguard, expressing their ideals.

    Altruism. Courage. Dignity. Creativity. Love. Humor. Gentleness. Pride. Compassion. Joy. Hope. Sensitivity. Honesty. Selflessness. Charity. Where do we put these intangibles in the systems hierarchy? Is the courage of a man who jumps into the Potomac a function of processes at the organ system level? Is bravery a matter of epinephrine, norepinephrine, and catecholamines? Is it mediated by axons, synaptic clefts, and storage granules? Certainly this must be part of the answer, but not all of it. Courage seems to be a matter of this and so much more. Is it experiences at the two-person system that are key? Something in the way this man was raised? Something taught to him of altruism by a mother or father or loving grandparent? No doubt. We are certain of it. But what more? Does he belong to a subculture that, despite our colossally narcissistic society, still condones sacrifice and selflessness? What are his religious convictions? For that matter, where *do* we put spiritual beliefs and longings in the systems hierarchy?

The truth is, we do not know where to place such intangibles. They do not fit neatly anywhere, yet they seem relevant everywhere. They are embedded in the essence of medicine, and we encounter them everywhere in our practice of it. Walk down the corridor of any hospital, and you will witness dramas unfolding that all pivot on intangibles. To the participants in those drama, the intangibles are everything. Our patients are not statistics, but people, struggling with the most profound and important events of their lives—events measured not by sodium concentrations and hematocrits, but by intangibles. Imagine 100 patients, 100 identical people with identical cancers of an identical organ (as though such were possible!). Imagine the pertinent enzymes are all elevated to identical levels. The radiographs cast identical worrisome lucencies on identical films of lung and brain. You would still be witnessing 100 vastly different human events. Each one of these "identical" people has had a different life, different values, different memories, hopes, dreams, partners, children, grandchildren, and friends. Each feels differently about pain, discouragement, fear, fighting on, or giving up. Histopathologically, perhaps, they are all nearly the same, but the essence of their struggles, defeats, triumphs, and setbacks is not found here. It is found in the intangibles. For each, the experience of life is unique. For each, it is comprised not of enzymes and cardiac glycosides, but of memories and ideals—our quest for meaning, our capacity for faith and love, our ability to trust and to accept solace, and, ultimately, it is comprised of the existential and spiritual underpinnings of our soul.

Clearly, modern medicine has tended to ignore these matters, although they are what is usually *most* on our patients' minds. Still, some argue the importance and significance of such concerns lie outside the purview of medicine proper. Some say these are issues for philosophers, perhaps for clergy. Some even assent such matters are personal, private—that doctors should not intrude. We believe, however, that *here* is a place where doctors can, indeed *must*, learn to feel comfortable and belong.

What to call these things? Where to put them? Throughout this book we have urged you to view patients from the perspective of the systems theory and the biopsychosocial model. Such a view broadens and deepens our understanding of human beings suffering from illness; it renders us more capable and better informed. In summary, it enables us to be more effective doctors. Beyond this, we believe a full understanding of our patients requires attention to the universalities, to the intangibles, to the existential nature of so much of what we do. Here it becomes as difficult as it is critical to find the right words. For some, religion explains what we are attempting to describe. Such people are comfortable with terms such as *God* and with such concepts as the *spirit* and *soul*. Yet others feel put off by such a vocabulary—people who still feel the power of these universalities and appreciate instinctively their immense importance. Many such people recoil from terms that have religious overtones. How do we find the words to express such matters to them? Finally, there are some who feel that all such considerations are antiscientific, inherently in opposition to the rational, analytical, empirical thrust of our Western scientific tradition. Such individuals are sincere, but we believe they fail to understand much of what medicine, and life, consist.

In the end, we find ourselves stymied. We cannot find the right words, but our experience in medicine has taught us not to reject what we still have failed to capture. We believe that, someday, someone will. The same yearning to capture the essence of the intangibles in life may have been on the mind of Walt Whitman when he wrote the following poem. It was first published in 1863 but was still being revised in 1881. Evidently, he had trouble finding the right words too.

> A noiseless patient spider,
> I mark'd where on a little promontory it stood isolated.
> Mark'd how to explore the vacant vast surrounding,
> It launch'd forth filament, filament, filament, out of itself,
> Ever unreeling them, ever tirelessly speeding them.
> And you O my soul where you stand,
> Surrounded, detached, in measureless oceans of space,
> Ceaselessly musing, venturing, throwing, seeking the spheres to connect them.
> Till the bridge you will need be form'd, till the ductile anchor hold,
> Till the gossamer thread you fling catch somewhere, O my soul.

## HEALING

There is a vast difference between curing and healing.[*,1] A patient can be cured but not healed. There are also many times when physicians can help patients to heal, although they cannot cure them. Sometimes, the latter opportunities provide the greatest joys and privileges physicians can hope to know. We close this chapter with such an example—the story of David, a little boy, and his family who were helped to heal by a deeply caring physician. The story of David is not ours. He was the patient of a very gifted and special doctor, Dr. Frances Sharkey. Her account of David is one of several in her superb book *A Parting Gift*,[8] a book that should be read by every medical student and every doctor who still has a longing to grow and learn.

David was a pale, taciturn 2½-year-old when pediatrician Dr. Sharkey first encountered him in her waiting room. He came accompanied by a brief referring note from his general practitioner. The note was only two words long. It read, "Hemoglobin 6." From

---

1 *To *cure* comes from the Latin word *curare* and means to take care of, to take charge of, and denotes successful medical treatment. To *heal* comes from the ancient English word *haelen* and means to make or become whole; it is closely related to the work *holy*, also derived from the same root.

the outset, Dr. Sharkey suspected leukemia, yet she was reluctant, as many physicians would be, to accept a diagnosis that seemed to extinguish hope:

> I patted the bruised little leg. How about a diagnosis of aplastic anemia? That wasn't a nice disease, but it could be treated and not prove fatal.
>
> One part of the baby remained to be examined before I could make even a provisional diagnosis in my mind of cancer or leukemia—a diagnosis that meant almost a death sentence for this beautiful child. I must feel his abdomen to see if his spleen is enlarged.
>
> I unbuttoned his shirt and look at his abdomen. It was fat like all 2-year-olds. Or was it fatter? I put my fingers on his chest. He bent his head and watched my hand. Soft skin, firm little ribs moving up and down with each breath. The pulsating of his heart was strong and normal. I ran my fingers downward. Then, light as was my touch, with no wince from the baby, I felt an enlarged spleen. (ref. 9)

From the outset, Dr. Sharkey related not only to David, but also to his parents. They did not warm up instantly to her; rather, the relationship grew and, over time, a powerful bond between them replaced shyness and distrust. Dr. Sharkey's relationship with Mr. and Mrs. Carver was marred early on, not by any lack of warmth, but by her initial misinterpretation of the medical facts. When David's leukemia was being diagnosed, the fields of hematology and oncology were changing so rapidly that most general pediatricians could not hope to keep up. Within several years, during the decade of the 1970s, acute lymphocytic leukemia (the form David had) ceased to be a uniformly fatal illness—truly a death sentence—and became a potentially curable disease. This astonishing biomedical progress has continued to this day. Now, children suffering from the disease are more likely to live than to die; but, initially, Dr. Sharkey knew none of this. She broke the painful "truth" to them, comforted them when they wept, and only later discovered she had been quite wrong. Her courage in admitting this mistake in the book, her willingness to share with her readers that she was fallible and human is one of the traits that makes Dr. Sharkey, and her book, so remarkable.

> Tears ran down Mrs. Carver's cheeks and she wiped them away with the back of her hand. I sat back and took my hand from hers. "There are good, effective drugs with which leukemia can be treated, at least for a while," I said.
>
> For the first time since I had sat down with them, she looked directly at me. Shock marred her young face. Her husband shifted uncomfortably in his chair. "How long—how long . . . ," he began. His voice faltered.
>
> "How long will he live?" I filled in for him. He nodded . . . .
>
> As physicians, we cannot witness illness and suffering in our patients so intensely without, on occasion, glimpsing intimations of our own mortality and that of the people we most dearly love.
>
> That night as I tucked my children into their beds, I put my hand on their abdomens and surreptitiously felt to see if any one of them had an enlarged spleen. It would be months before I lost the need to reassure myself they didn't.

David responded well to the drugs administered to reverse his acute crisis. Color returned to his face, liveliness and vitality to his play. Dr. Sharkey was soon able to send him home. There is a passage in the book at this point that captures, for us, the essence of medicine as a human experience. Dr. Sharkey is talking with David's parents before his discharge. What she has to say makes it clear that it is never a matter of "either" humanism "or" science. It is, inevitably, an amalgam of both.

"There's another way therapy has been improved just recently. Although it's new, I want David to have it—radiation to his brain . . . ."

I already did a spinal tap on David and injected methotrexate into his spinal fluid. That also decreases the chance of malignant cells growing around his brain. The spinal tap wasn't painful, but he had to be held tightly, which scares most children. Not David! He cried for a minute and then quieted down and just lay trustingly in the arms of the nurse. He's a wonderfully calm baby.

Mrs. Carver nodded her head and kissed David's cheek lightly.

"Here," I said, reaching into my bag and bringing out a sheaf of journal articles, "these are for you to read. The past few days I've reviewed the literature on leukemia. It's marvelously encouraging and speaks of 50 percent cure rates with current therapy."

I handed Mr. Carver copies of the articles I had read. "A week ago I said that David's disease was fatal. I hadn't read up on leukemia then. My statement may already be out of date. I certainly hope it is."

"You can take David home . . . ."

In the ensuing months, Dr. Sharkey assumed responsibility for all parts of David's treatment. Instead of sending him to a specialist for his anticancer drugs, she consulted the specialists but administered the treatments herself. With each office visit, David seemed to grow stronger—and with his physical rebirth, hope, too, began to thrive:

Safe in his mother's arms David regarded me with wide eyes. "He's 2½ years old, I thought." In 5 years, if he lives, he'll be in the second grade. Could that be possible? Would I be saying to these parents someday in the future, "David is cured . . . ."

So, too, did the relationship between Dr. Sharkey and the Carvers deepen and thrive:

Mr. Carver shook hands with me. The contact of our hands was firm and reassuring. Mrs. Carver smiled as if I were an old friend. She held David in her arms.

"He doesn't say many words yet but I've taught him your name. Come on, David," she coaxed, "You know it."

David looked shy and then, knowing how much it would please her, he flung his chubby arms up and said, "Docta Shark."

Months blended into years. David's response to the radiation treatment was good, and there were no further signs of leukemia. He and his family began to feel that perhaps, just maybe, they were not treasuring life under the shadow of death. Mrs. Carver soon became pregnant.

David lived to enter kindergarten, then first grade. Both passed without incident. The little boy Dr. Sharkey once thought doomed to die was now an active, rambunctious 6-year-old asserting to his father that the training wheel just had to come off his bicycle, that instant! When David came to Dr. Sharkey's office now it was with pride, and just a hint of a boyish flirt, that he pulled off his shirt and flexed his biceps for her.

Finally, after 5 years of chemotherapy, the time had come to stop David's medication. Taking him off the drugs was a huge step. Everyone wondered what might happen after they relinquished David's now-familiar and reassuring chemical safety net. However, as a consultant had correctly remarked, "We can't keep him on the drugs forever." Dr. Sharkey and David's parents realized they must find the courage to let go.

The drugs were stopped. David remained well. Dr. Sharkey began to cut back from the schedule of weekly office visits. He seemed cured, and it was time to let him leave the medical nest.

When David turned 8, however, tragedy struck. Dr. Sharkey discovered it during a routine physical:

> I ran my hands over David's familiar body. He was, despite the radiation therapy and drugs, a big child. Recently his body shape had matured and his muscles were chunkier. As usual, at the end of the exam I felt his testes. David no longer giggled the way he had when he was younger but tolerated this patiently. All at once I was alarmed. Was I imagining it or did his testes feel larger? There were no hard lumps and there was nothing irregular about them, but they definitely had increased in size.

Because leukemia of this type was most apt to recur in the testes or brain, the finding was frightening. It also posed very difficult decisions regarding what should be done at that point. No discrete mass in the testes had been found, but by the time a mass was found it might be too late. The question she struggled with was should they irradiate his testes immediately? It might be effective, but it would sterilize David for life. He was 8; the growth of his testes *could* be early enlargement prior to puberty. Should anyone risk sterilizing David just on the *chance* that his leukemia might recur? Either way, they had to play a fearsome game of Russian roulette with David's life and future at stake. They decided not to irradiate.

Several months later, the time bomb exploded. Dr. Sharkey had just returned from a trip to India. She had gone in to the hospital to make rounds on a hospitalized child. She was sitting at the nurses' station:

> As I sat there, an intern and a resident came by making their evening rounds. They were discussing each patient briefly.

"Welcome back," one said. "You've got Theresa's chart. She did really well while you were gone. She even gets up and walks to physical therapy now."

Leaving me, they went on to talk about the next patient. Although I was reading Theresa's chart I could hear their words.

"In this room is a child with leukemia in relapse."

Suddenly Theresa's chart felt as if it weighed a hundred pounds. Unconsciously I held my breath, waiting for their next words.

"Whose patient is it?" the resident asked the intern.

It was David.

The prospect now was very depressing. When leukemia had recurred only in the testes, the literature indicated a fighting chance. When it had recurred only in the bone marrow, there was also still hope for a cure; but if malignancy was discovered in both sites, the odds of a child's living more than a year were virtually nonexistent. This is what had happened to David.

Heroic efforts nevertheless continued. New drug protocols were coming out all the time, and with courage and fierce hope Dr. Sharkey fought on, struggling to find the magic combination of drugs and irradiation that might still offer David a chance.

In the end, it was a fight she lost. Now, not only did she feel the anguish and pain of her own grief, Dr. Sharkey also struggled to find the right words to say to David and his family.

David now came to my office once a week. He'd gone to school a few times, but it tired him badly. He looked so ill his classmates were frightened. We arranged for a home teacher to come to his house every day. She asked me how much work she should give him. Did I ever expect him to rejoin his class?

"No," I said sadly, "but he must continue with his schoolwork. Taking it away from him would be like telling him he was going to die."

Now when he came into the office, he needed my help to climb onto the examining-room table. He was embarrassed by his weakness. In his thin face his smile had lost none of its sweetness.

He knew his disease was back, and he knew it was leukemia. I wondered if he had ever seen a television program about anyone dying from leukemia. I wondered if he thought this was happening to him. I hadn't said anything to him about dying. For that matter, I hadn't said anything to his parents, either.

With the reality of David's death now a certainty, Dr. Sharkey also had to relive the misery she had experienced when other children had died. Many of these deaths had been painful and terrifying. Worse still, they had come in a hospital, with the anguished child separated from his parents when he needed them most. Hospitals, Dr. Sharkey was beginning to think, were *not* where children should have to die. In the hospital, children tended to die alone—and their parents suffered alone. Dr. Sharkey began to wonder: Was this really in the name of optimal patient care? Or had the elaborate system of rules, regulations, protocol, and hospital routine actually been erected to protect the staff from the pain *they* might feel if the struggles of these children and their families suddenly became too real?

> Late one afternoon I asked Betty and Stan to come to my office. Finally, I had to tell them there was no hope; there was nothing further I could do for David. Until that was said, there was no way we could plan for his death. I was terribly depressed. By admitting that there was nothing more I could do for David, I felt I was no longer needed. Yet on a deeper level I realized I was needed more than ever.
>
> We sat in front of the window in my office for a few minutes and watched the shadows lengthen on the hills. I finally broke the silence. "David gets closer to death each day. I've said nothing to him about dying. I must soon. I've always been uncomfortable watching the children who die in the hospital. It seems to me that children hate being in the hospital and would be much more at peace in their own homes. Before I tell David he's dying, I want to know what your feelings are about where he should die."
>
> Betty reached out for her husband's hand. Tears filled her eyes. "We want David where it is best for him . . . . We'll keep him at home . . . ."

Dr. Sharkey now had to endure a tremendous outpouring of defensiveness and disapproval from her colleagues. Her natural tenderness, open expressions of love and affection—all these had already led some uneasy colleagues to accuse her of being "overly involved" of "losing professional detachment." Her decision to send David home was more than most of them could bear. They accused her of losing all sense of professional responsibility. She was upbraided for not giving *every* new regimen on the horizon a try. More than one physician came close to accusing her of depriving David of a chance for cure. When Dr. Sharkey held her ground, colleagues finally shrugged their shoulders and said, "Well, it's your case," thus isolating her and ensuring she would feel alone and unsupported.

We can only imagine the loneliness and pain she had to endure at the hands of "colleagues." Already she suffered deeply at David's impending death. She was trying to help his family. Surely, she, too, now needed all the support and empathy her colleagues could offer. Instead, she was ostracized: "It's your patient." The message was clear: If you want to confront what we're afraid of, we'll push you away. You'll do it on your own.

What a lonely path she was forced to take for doing what she believed was right:

> Time was running out.
> I took his frail body in my arms and cradled his head against me.
> "David, most of the time when we're sick, we take medicine and it makes us better. But sometimes the medicine doesn't work and we don't get well. We die." I felt his body tense. I held him closely and rocked him as if he were a baby. "I'm going to die someday, and your mommy is going to die someday, too. Usually mommies die before their children, but sometimes . . . sometimes . . . ." My voice failed

me. I kissed the top of his head and saw my tears fall on his hair. His arms were around me. He tightened them as he nestled closer.

"Am I going to die?" he asked, his voice muffled against me.

"Yes, David."

"Does my mommy know?"

"Yes, and John and your daddy know, even Mary. They want you at home with them."

"Will it hurt?" asked this child who had never let us know he was frightened.

"No, I don't think so. It'll just be like going to sleep. And your mommy will be with you."

We held each other in a profound silence. I realized with wonder that what I had said had not shocked him at all. Why had I waited so long, making excuses to myself that I needed the perfect moment? There is no such thing as the perfect moment. We make all our moments, and by the truth and love we bring to them, we make them perfect. David had probably thought he was dying for at least a month, maybe longer. His innate sensitivity had made him keep that from us.

My arms were cramped. "Is there anything you want?" I asked, shifting his weight.

"Would you rub my back?" he said. "It hurts."

I couldn't save him, and I couldn't tell him what death was like. But I could rub his back.

Finally, the day came for his discharge from the hospital.

The next morning when I entered David's room, the intravenous line had been disconnected. The heparin lock was neatly taped in place on his hand.

"Are you actually discharging him?" asked the resident doctor.

"Yes."

"And his mother is going to treat his bloodstream infection? Isn't that asking a bit much of her?"

I didn't answer him.

"Why don't you keep him here a few weeks and treat him properly for the infection?" he persisted.

"Because he doesn't have a few weeks," I snapped. "He'll be treated just as properly at home as in the hospital. Does it matter whether a nurse or his mother injects the antibiotic? But even if we could clear up the bloodstream infection, it wouldn't save his life. If he doesn't go home today, I'm afraid he'll never go home again."

"He's your patient," the resident said sarcastically and walked away.

I wrote the discharge order. David, wrapped in a blanket, was carried out of the hospital in his father's arms.

Every day Dr. Sharkey visited David. One of her own children, aware of how absorbed her mother had become with this mysterious dying boy, also groped to understand. Finally, Dr. Sharkey's daughter went and fetched a book of poems, tattered from use, and gave it to her mother to read to David. It was her favorite book.

That afternoon, Dr. Sharkey read David the poems from her daughter's book while David smiled and lay curled in her arms.

As time went on, David grew very weak and ill.

I leaned over him. His breathing was rapid. His face was warm with fever. I sat beside him and listened to his chest with my stethoscope. My touch awakened him. He looked at me with recognition and smiled weakly. I stroked his hair. "Do you want a poem?" I asked softly. He nodded and closed his eyes.

I sat with my arm around him and read him a very short one. He didn't seem to be listening. "Do you want another poem?" I asked. He shook his head and closed his eyes. I put my cheek against his and then kissed him.

Here is the closing passage from the book:

On Saturday morning when Stan was home from work David awakened, once again inexplicably interested in his surroundings. He got out of the big bed and went to the bathroom and then walked back to his own bed in the dining room. He lay down but didn't fall asleep. Betty was surprised by this and heartened by the fact that he was up again. She'd scarcely left his side for 3 days. She thought, "He's so alert, he can't possibly die right now." She kissed him on his forehead and asked, "Is it all right if I go shopping for a little while?" He touched her hand and nodded his head. She noticed that his dark eyes seemed more beautiful than ever. She left, anxious to get the shopping over with and be back with him.

David lay on his bed and looked out of the window. He could see his sister playing on the front lawn. The kitten was on the windowsill, trying to catch a fly.

After a little while David asked his father for some morphine. He swallowed a spoonful and made a face. He asked for some juice. Stan went to the kitchen to get some from the refrigerator. He could see David all the time. David was lying on his back on the bed. He held his hands in front of his face, looking at them. He stretched out his arms and then brought his hands in close to his eyes. He seemed to be examining each finger the way a baby does when it first discovers its hands.

Stan turned his attention to pouring the juice. When he brought it to the bed, David was dead.

David hadn't made a sound. His father couldn't believe it. He sat by David, almost expecting him to breathe again. David's eyes were closed. He looked as if he had just fallen asleep.

Stan sat by David awhile and then went outside and called Mary and John. The two children went to the bed where the body of their dead brother lay. Mary ran her finger along David's arm and put her head down next to his on the pillow. John stood looking at David and then went to the window and picked up the kitten. He brought the kitten to the bed and curled it up next to David, placing his dead brother's arms around the kitten in the position it had rested so often.

When Betty came home that was how she found her family.

Is this painful? Yes. Excruciatingly so. Yet it is also excruciatingly beautiful. It is healing just to read it.

Every student should read Dr. Sharkey's book. It is a masterpiece. Suffice it to say here, the book is about far more than death, although it is certainly about this, too. It is about love, courage, altruism, mystery, and awe—the human essence of our work. Although it is painful to touch on these things, in the end, it is only by fleeing from them that we ourselves will fail to heal.

Medicine *is* a human experience, propelled forward by science but guided by love.

## REFERENCES

1. Bosworth A. Nuclear weapons pose greater threat than climate change. *Cornell Chronicle*. February 11, 2016. http://www.news.cornell.edu/stories/2016/02/nuclear-weapons-pose-greater-threat-climate-change. Accessed August 14, 2016.
2. Shanafelt TD, Hasan O, Dyrbye LN, et al. Changes in burnout and satisfaction with work–life balance in physicians and the general US working population between 2011 and 2014. *Mayo Clin Proc*. 2015;90(12):1600–1613.
3. Ariely D, Lanier WL. Disturbing trends in physician burnout and satisfaction with work–life balance: dealing with malady among the nation's healers. *Mayo Clin Proc*. 2015;90(12):1593–1596.
4. National Center for Complementary and Integrative Health. *The Use of Complementary and Alternative Medicine in the United States*. National Institutes of Health. December 2008. https://nccih.nih.gov/research/statistics/2007/camsurvey_fs1.htm. Accessed August 14, 2016.
5. Thomas L. *The Youngest Science: Notes of a Medicine-Watcher*. New York: Viking Press; 1983:55–60.
6. Lynch JJ. *The Broken Heart: The Medical Consequences of Loneliness*. New York: Basic Books, 1977.
7. Malraux A. *Man's Fate*. New York: Harrison Smith & Robert Haas; 1934.
8. Sharkey F. *A Parting Gift*. New York: St. Martin's Press; 1982.

## SUGGESTED READINGS

Boyd W. *The Spontaneous Regression of Cancer*. Springfield, IL: Charles C. Thomas; 1966.

Cassell EJ. The nature of suffering and the goals of medicine. *N Engl J Med*. 1982;306:639–645.

Cousins N. *Anatomy of an Illness as Perceived by the Patient: Reflections on Healing and Regeneration*. New York: Norton; 1979.

Cousins N. *The Healing Heart: Antidotes to Panic and Helplessness*. New York: Norton; 1983.

Rosen DH. Casualties of the health care system: patients depressed by medicine: moral dilemmas. *Pharos*. 1987;50:19–20.

Rosen DH. *Lost in the Long White Cloud: Finding My Way Home: Conception Through the Death of My Father*. Eugene: Wipf & Stock Publishers; 2014

Rosen DH. The Tao of medicine. *Pharos*. 2000;63:14.

Rosen DH, Blackwell B. Teaching psychiatry in medicine: the development of a unique clinical course. *Arch Intern Med*. 1982;142:113–115.

Rosen DH, Weishaus J. *The Healing Spirit of Haiku*. Eugene: Resource Publications (a division of Wipf & Stock Publishers); 2014.

Tumulty PA. The art of healing. *Johns Hopkins Med J*. 1978;143:140–143.

Weiss PA. Causality: linear or systemic. In: *Psychology and Biology of Language and Thought*. New York: Academic Press; 1978:13–26.

# EPILOGUE: DESIDERATA

During the 16th century in England, an anonymous individual carved a series of desiderata in a wooden church door. They were apparently offered as guides to young novitiates on how to lead effective, harmonious lives. During the 1960s and 1970s, these desiderata were rediscovered and circulated widely on posters that found their way onto many walls. Centuries later, the world is still in colossal turmoil, and the desiderata still make sense. The lyricism and wisdom of the desiderata are, in fact, remarkable. There is so much beauty in them that even repeated reading discloses something fresh and new.

What we offer here is far more modest. Our desiderata are short and to the point. However, we felt it appropriate somehow to close this book with some "words of wisdom" to the young men and women we are attempting to teach, who have embraced the impossibilities of this fascinating and excruciating calling.

*Remember that being a doctor is a privilege.* When you face the trauma and savagery that humans can inflict on fellow humans, that life sometimes inflicts on us all, when you see human beings reduced to an ugliness that you once thought unimaginable; when you see doctors, nurses, and even yourself treating people with a callousness you once never dreamed would be possible—remember, you are privileged. It is true that doctors are no longer held in blind esteem by the general public. This is for the better. But, you remain part of a powerful, respected, and protected profession. Certainly there are financial rewards, but the privilege is really a much deeper one. By your choice of calling, you have been invited to be a trusted and intimate participant in the most elemental and basic moments of human life: birth, death, regeneration, decline; madness, pain, and instances of unbelievable clarity. Very few will ever be so permitted or so graced. You have been granted communion with life's most important mysteries. Artists and priests go where you go, but they lack your knowledge and skills to help scientifically. On the other hand, do not ignore their capacity to see beauty where others see only the mundane or ugly. Learn the poet's appreciation for human nobility and transcendent spirit. It is within your reach. When your privilege begins to feel like a burden—and at times it will—remember how fortunate you are to live life so fully.

*Remember that you are free.* There are few professions in which one is as free to choose as medicine. You can go to the National Institutes of Health and study AIDS. You can go to Native American reservations to treat the underserved. It is all up to you. Your education confers a staggering number of options, yet medical school education is so often hierarchical, constrictive, and authoritarian that students lose sight of this. Sadly, by graduation time many new doctors have forgotten what it means to be free, even after the chains and shackles have been removed. This is the saddest tyranny of all.

If enough young physicians remember they are free, there will come a true renaissance in medicine; many different styles and kinds of practice will flourish and coexist. We will no longer be so distrusted and envied as a profession. It must be said, that at times, our wealth, power, and privilege do seem to be excessive and unreasonable, especially in a world so full of suffering, deprivation, hunger, and want. In the end, however, only our own failure to remember that we are free will cause us to go the way of the dinosaur. This seems very unlikely to happen. Mostly, it rests with you, the next generation of physicians.

*Empathize with the plight of your fellow professionals.* When your resident dumps on you, when the nurses are cold, when the attending humiliates you, when you see people treating patients like castoffs instead of human beings—remember they are really only people too, like yourself. They are struggling with the same questions, torments, and responsibilities you are. Have compassion, especially for the house staff. Their pressures await you. The demands are awesome, and the help these young doctors get is varied and can be limited.

*Remember why you decided to be a doctor.* If you are like most of us, you did not choose medicine solely to do pure research, and it certainly was not to own a huge home on the first tee of the golf course. Remember, too, as you are being trained in an academic setting, that you did not necessarily choose medicine to be famous and important. You chose medicine because you are interested in healing the mind, body, and spirit, and because—as sentimental as it sounds—you care about people. Remember this when someone humiliates you for not knowing everything about everything. Keep it in mind when you are tempted to recoil from patients who seem ravaged beyond hope, almost beyond human recognition. You chose medicine because you care.

*Medical school does not last forever.* This is difficult to remember sometimes, but it is true. If you are a junior, your formal education will average another 6 years. This is a long time, but it is not forever. Remember the human, gentle qualities you cherish in yourself and that seem to go underground during these years. You may fear, at times, these traits are lost hopelessly forever. However, be assured, they can and do come back. Do not be overly discouraged, either, by the sometimes callous behavior of house officers; their struggles are huge. Do not be overly impressed or dismayed by your academic teachers. Teachers are important, and we need them. Medicine needs researchers and scholars as well. Sometimes, too often perhaps, the academicians who teach you are people who have failed to grow up in some ways. They remain "in training" forever—always climbing the ladder of success, always competing, always conscious of the hierarchy. Do not let their mockery of the practicing physician dissuade you. Certainly private medicine has its share of incompetents. So does academic medicine. There are many wise, happy, and mature doctors in both settings, as well. Seek out the role models you respect for both their knowledge and the care they provide. Hold on to the realistic conviction that you can get there eventually.

*Forgive yourself.* Just as you should forgive those around you, learn early to forgive yourself. You will make mistakes. You will do terrible things—not as often as you fear, but now and again. You will fail to be perfect. You will blunder technically and, on occasion, your sadism toward patients may shock and depress you. However, this is a line of work filled with impossibilities. Show yourself generosity and compassion. It will make you a better doctor for your patients as well.

*Accept ambiguity and personal limitations.* Despite our wish for certainty, medicine is and will always remain an ambiguous field. Those who think that science will ultimately eliminate this ambiguity are dreamers. The more our science advances, the more fundamental and deeply vexing the ambiguities we face will become. If you cannot learn to tolerate ambiguity in medicine—and it is very difficult for most of us—your life as a doctor will be filled with torment. If you can learn to accept ambiguity, you will see beauty and splendor where others see only disorder and frustration. Accept your own limitations. You cannot know everything. You cannot do everything. You cannot be everything. Some people will be better at some things than you. You will never gain full mastery. Ever. Accept this, and peace will replace frustration and fear. Refuse to accept it, and you will drive yourself into a life of pettiness, envy, and despair. Do not be afraid to draw boxes. We all do. We must. It is fun to have a little corner where things are less ambiguous and where our mastery, relatively speaking, is greater. However, beware of people who draw boxes, pretend that everything inside those boxes is certain, and denigrate what lies beyond the perimeters of their own narrow conceits. Keep your eyes peeled. Watch out especially for any doctors who put other doctors down just because they are different.

*Physician, heal thyself.* There is growing concern over the dehumanizing and fragmented nature of medical practice. Most of the attention has focused on the destructive effects this has on the patient. The emergence of such concern is appropriate and heartening. The title of this book reflects our conviction that our experiences in medicine must be human and humane. This includes our patients and ourselves, but as a group, we—doctors—have been curiously, and often tragically, neglected. There is a growing awareness of the severity and prevalence of physician impairment. Suicide. Alcoholism. Drug addiction. You have all heard the statistics—and do not say it could never happen to you, because it could. A number of these 8 desiderata were constructed with just this concern in mind. No book can replace a humane and informed system of education. On the other hand, we seriously doubt if any physician truly could follow the spirit of these 8 desiderata and become impaired. Full of hurt, in need of help—yes; but hopelessly isolated and alone, devastatingly impaired? We doubt it. Beyond this, we are just as concerned about "unimpaired physicians," the driven, workaholic perfectionists who cannot unwind or have fun, who never see their family and seem likely candidates for a heart attack. A pillar of the community, they are hardly impaired. Yet we fear they may be lost—so much of the joy and wonder of medicine seems to elude them. Physicians who become alcoholics or addicted are a tragedy, but they are only the tip of an awesome iceberg. It is an equally sad fact that too few physicians are actually very happy. You would be surprised to learn how widespread this unhappiness really is. This is terrible, for our calling offers so much potential for growth, creativity, beauty, and meaning. Something clearly is wrong with the way we are educating doctors. It is a complicated problem, with origins in realms as diverse as the knowledge explosion, economics, and politics. We have no wish to oversimplify the problem, but we are convinced that a major source of physician unhappiness lies in the lack of compassion and empathy with which we treat ourselves. We are not talking here about anything as simple as overly demanding call schedules (although we are talking about that too). We are talking about a more silent yet malignant view of physicianhood that ignores, indeed attacks, the rights and needs of physicians themselves to be sensitive, to feel pain, to be human beings. Doctors are taught and then reinforced in countless ways that they should hold feelings in, go it alone, never let their vulnerability show. Never, it seems, should one reach out, express vulnerability, experience and permit human needs. No wonder doctors are so poor at permitting these same vital needs to emerge in their patients! When this kind of socialization becomes coupled with other traits so common to physicians—a driving perfectionism, unforgivingly high self-standards, a tremendous need for mastery and control—then we have a situation that is very dangerous. For every addicted physician, there are a hundred unhappy workaholics. For every suicide, there are a thousand quietly lonely, vaguely depressed doctors who do a wonderful job with their patients but somehow never get to see their children grow up, never experience deep love and peace. These are doctors who wonder too late, "Where did my life go? What did it all mean?"

Although the issue is admittedly complex, we believe that ultimate revolution in medical education will come from within. We must begin to nurture the needs, hopes, and sensitivities of the promising young men and women who have elected to adopt this unique, stressful, beautiful, and perilous career. We must encourage introspection, healthy relationships, play, openness, and joyous, creative expression. We must spawn a generation of doctors who are not afraid to love.

# INDEX

AAMC. *See* Association of American Medical Colleges
acceptance, 5–8, 15, 21–24
   healing and, 108, 116, 123–24
   illness and, 92
Accreditation Council for Graduate Medical Education (ACGME), 3
acetazolamide, 17
ACGME. *See* Accreditation Council for Graduate Medical Education
acquired immune deficiency syndrome (AIDS), 139
acute bacterial endocarditis, 103
addiction, drug, 82, 141
affect, in doctor-patient relations, 71–72
AIDS. *See* acquired immune deficiency syndrome
alcoholism, 9, 20–21, 82, 141
altitude sickness, 16–19
altruism, 126–28, 137
ambiguity, 15, 23–24, 140–41
ambivalence, 89–90
American Board of Medical Specialties, 3
amyotrophic lateral sclerosis, 93
anxiety
   awareness of illness and, 89–90
   in doctor-patient relations, 61–63
apology, 84–85
arterial puncture, 36–38, 37*f*
A.R.T. paradigm, 74–79
Association of American Medical Colleges (AAMC), 3–4
attitude, 5–8. *See also* illness
authenticity, 80
awareness, 7, 24. *See also* illness
   in doctor-patient relationship, 87–95
   in illness, 100
   meditation and, 19, 81, 110–11, 120, 125
   mortality and, 89–92

Balint, Michael, 56–57
barium enema, 55
bedside manner, 7, 28, 53, 55, 66, 88, 108. *See also* doctor-patient relationship
Bertalanffy, Ludwig von, 29
biomedical model
   biopsychosocial model comparison of, 36–42, 37*f*, 39*f*–41*f*
   as dogma, 39–42
   in hierarchy of systems, 27–29
   limits of, 27–29
biomolecular technology, 14
biopsychosocial model, xix–xx
   application of, 31–36, 33*f*, 35*f*
   biomedical model comparison to, 36–42, 37*f*, 39*f*–41*f*
   counter-dogma of, 40–42
   in doctor-patient relations, 58–61
   Engel and, 13, 15–16, 19–20
   healing and, 123–26
   interviewing in, 69–79
   MCAT and, 4
   in medical paradigm shift, 4
   medical student and, 57–60
   nervous system in, 29, 30*f*, 31*f*, 34–36
   person-level factors in, 33–38, 35*f*
   in systems hierarchy, 29–31, 30*f*, 31*f*
   in treatment strategies, 49–51
biopsychosocialspiritual model, ix. *See also* integrative medicine
biosphere, 19–20
body language, 45–49, 80–83
burnout, 59, 110

cancer, reorganization and, 92–93
cardiac arrest, 36–38, 39*f*
   in Type A personality, 48–51
Cartesian dualism, 66, 125–26
Cassem, Ned, 7

cell, 29, 30f, 31f, 109
central toxic keratopathy (CTK), 23–24
children, 6–7, 46–47, 63. *See also* human development
codeine, 89
communication. *See also* doctor-patient relationship
   interview process in, 72–74
   in medicine, xi–xv
   nonverbal language in, 45–49
   observation in, 69–71
   repeating last words in, 82
   verbal language in, 53–56
compassion, 18–19, 140
   example of, 23–24
   medical student and, 58–59
compensation patient, 105
competency, 20–24, 109
conceptualization, 13–20. *See also* illness
confidentiality, 80
congestive heart failure, 47–48, 69–70, 104
coping, 100–103
corporate healthcare. *See* healthcare system
counseling, psychological, xvi, 89
countertransference, 64–65
Cousins, Norman, xv
Crohn's disease, 84
*Crossing the Quality Chasm: A New Health System for 21st Century* (IOM), 2
crying, 80–81
CTK. *See* central toxic keratopathy
curing. *See* healing
curiosity, 58
cyanide, 126

death. *See also* suicide
   denial of, 66–67, 89–91
   *A Parting Gift* story and, 129–37
defense mechanisms, 101–2
defensiveness, 12, 83, 123, 134
defibrillation, 38, 40f–41f
dehumanization, xx, 2, 67, 141
denial, 66–67, 89–91
depression, 60–61, 64, 88, 102. *See also* illness
desiderata, 139–42
developmental psychology, 6–7
diabetes, 9, 56, 87, 92, 97–98

diagnostic interview. *See also* doctor-patient relationship
   affect in, 71–72
   A.R.T. paradigm in, 74–79
   assessment in, 76–78
   observation in, 69–71
   process of, 72–74
   ranking in, 78
   transition in, 78–79
   visual skills in, 69–71
diffuse lamellar keratitis, 23
disorganization, illness and, 90–92
doctor-patient relationship. *See also* patient-centered care
   affect in, 71–72
   anxiety in, 61–63
   awareness in, 87–95
   in challenges of illness, 99–100
   compassion in, 58–59
   cultural background in, 27
   in curing and healing, 107–11
   curiosity in, 58
   empathy in, 8–13, 53–54, 61–63, 108–9
   Engel and, 57, 59, 61, 63, 66, 69
   feelings in, 63–67
   interview process in, 72–74
   language in, 53–56
   medical student in, 57–60
   new trends in, 14
   *A Parting Gift* story of, 129–37
   patient examples of, 111–20
   personal style in, 59
   power of, 56–57
   responsibility in, 59–60
   shamanism and, 67, 121
   slang in, 65–66
   touching and, 120–23
   Type A personality in, 48–51
dogma, of biomedical model, 39–42
Dolly the sheep, 14
drug addiction, 82, 141
dualism, 27–29, 66

Eisenberg, Leon, 104
empathy
   in biopsychosocial approach, xx
   breakdown in, 9
   in curing and healing, 108–9

between healthcare providers, 140
language and, 53–54
objective reality in, 12
in patient anxiety, 61–63
as principle, 8–13
empty nest syndrome, 62
endocrine system. *See also* biopsychosocial model
panic and stress in, xiv–xv, 23
Engel, George, xix–xx, 4
biopsychosocial model of, 13, 15–16, 19–20
in doctor-patient relations, 57, 59, 61, 63, 66, 69
Giving-up/Given-up Complex and, 98–99
observational skills and, 69
Erikson, Erik, 62
expectations, management of, 84. *See also* illness

facial expression, 45–46, 70, 82
family doctor, ix, 14–16
fatal grief, 95–99
fatigue, 16–19
feelings. *See also* illness
affect of, 71–72
countertransference of, 64–65
denial of death and, 66–67, 89–91
fatal grief and, 95–99
slang in, 65–66
transference of, 64–65
forgiveness, 140
Fox, Terry, 127
Freud, Sigmund, 76
Friedman, Meyer, 48
Frost, Robert, 15, 24

Gates, Bill, 22
Gehrig, Lou, 93
gene-editing technology, 14
general practitioner (GP), ix, 14–16
generosity, 140
Giving-up/Given-up Complex, 98–99
Goldman, Brian, 84
Good, Byron, 104
GP. *See* general practitioner
*Graduate Medical Education That Meets Nation's Health Needs* (IOM), 3

guided visual imagery, 116–20
Gull, Sir William, 51

Hackett, Thomas, 7
headache, 14, 88–89
healing. *See also* illness
biopsychosocial model, 123–26
distinction between curing and, 107–11
empathy in, 108–9
*A Parting Gift* story and, 129–37
patient examples of, 111–20
process of, 85
touching and, 120–23
visualization in, 116–20
healthcare system. *See also* patient-centered care
ambiguity in, 140–41
dehumanizing in, xx, 2, 67, 141
disappointment with, 123–26
economic crisis of, ix
Latin terms in, ix, 5, 129
Health Insurance Portability and Accountability Act, 80
*Health Professions Education: A Bridge to Quality* (IOM), 2
health-seeking behavior, 88–89
*Heartsounds* (Lear), 95
Helfand, Ira, 109
helplessness, 44–45
in conceptualization, 16–19
nonverbal gesture of, 45–47
hematuria, 87
Hertzog, Leif, 21–24
hierarchy of systems, 13–14, 19–20
biomedical model in, 27–29
biopsychosocial model in, 29–31, 30*f*, 31*f*
molecular substance in, 30–31, 30*f*, 31*f*
stable configuration of, 29
stages of illness and, 87–89
Hippocrates, 2
Hippocratic oath, 80
Hoang, Uyen, xx, 16–19, 21, 80, 107–8
holistic medicine, 124–26 *See also* biopsychosocial model
hope, in terminal illness, 95–99

hospitalization. *See also* illness
  dehumanization in, xx, 2, 67, 141
  emergency room and, 36, 50, 87
  holistic medicine and, 124–26
  medical slang in, 65–66
  patient feelings of, 62–63
  "problem patients" and, 104–5
  stages of illness and, 87–95
human development
  infant-parent relations in, 6–7, 46–47, 63, 109
  stages of illness and, 87–89
human spirit, xi, 24, 139–40
  interdependency and, 13–16
humor, 71, 80
hypochondriasis, 90

iatrogenic complications, xiii–xv, 20
identity diffusion, 110
illness
  awareness in, 89–90
  challenges of, 99–100
  Chinese symbol for, 87
  coping in, 100–103
  disorganization in, 90–92
  experience of, 87, 95–99
  "problem" patients and, 104–5
  reorganization in, 92–95
  stages of, 87–89
infant-parent relations, 6–7, 46–47, 63, 109
Institute of Medicine (IOM), 2–3
integrative medicine, ix. *See also* biopsychosocial model
  principles of, xi–xvii
International Physicians for Prevention of Nuclear War, 109
interpersonal transaction, 43–45
  nonverbal communication in, 45–49
  of Type A personality, 48–51
interviewing. *See* doctor-patient relationship; patient-centered interview
IOM. *See* Institute of Medicine

Kaiser Family Foundation, xix
Keller, Helen, 93
Keniston, Kenneth, 67
Kleinman, Arthur, 104
Kopacz, David, 101

language
  in curing and healing, 109–10
  in doctor-patient relations, 53–56
  nonverbal, 45–49, 80–83
  tone in, 71
laser-assisted in situ keratomileusis (LASIK), 21–24
Latin terms, ix, 5, 129
Lear, Martha W., 95–97
leukemia, 90, 113, 130–33
Levinson, Daniel, 62, 81
linear causality, 29
listening, skill of, 7–8
  lack of, 14–15
litigation, fear of, 85
llamas, 98
loneliness, xvii, 62, 82, 100, 119, 123, 134
lumbar puncture, 54
Lynch, James, 122

malignant melanoma, 116–17
Malraux, Andre, 126
*Man's Fate* (Malraux), 126
maternal acceptance, 6–7
Medical College Admissions Test (MCAT), 3–4
medical school, 140
medical student
  biopsychosocial perspective of, 57–58
  compassion of, 58–59
  curiosity of, 58
  insecurity of, 11–12
  MCAT and, 3–4
  observation and, 69–71
  *A Parting Gift* story and, 129
  in patient-centered care, 14–15, 50–51
  in patient-centered interview, 75, 80–84
  patient examples and, 111–20
  personal style of, 59
  responsibility and, 59–60
  slang and, 65–66
  stages of illness and, 89–90, 93, 98
Medicare, 54
medicine, principles of. *See* principles of medicine
*Medicine as a Human Experience* (Reiser and Rosen), xi–xii, xix, 1–2
meditation, 19, 81, 110–11, 120, 125

melanoma, 116–17
migraine headaches, 14, 88–89
Miller, B. J., 66
mistakes, in therapeutic relations, 84–85
Moliere, 121
Montaigne, Michel, 121, 124
Moos, Rudolf, 99, 102
morbid obesity, 60–61, 64
mortality, xvii, 66–67
    awareness and, 89–92
multiple sclerosis, 93
myocardial infarction, 32–38, 33*f*, 35*f*, 49, 93

National Center for Complementary and Integrative Health, 110
National Institute of Health, 139
nervous system, in biopsychosocial model, 29, 30*f*, 31*f*, 34–36
Newton, Isaac, 27
nihilism, 66, 94
nonverbal language, 45–49, 80–83

obesity, 60–61, 64
objective reality, 12
observation, in patient-centered interview, 69–71
omnipotence, 91–92
open-endedness, 77–78
ophthalmology, 21–24
opioids, 14
*Optimizing: A Five-Year Road Map for America's Medical Schools, Teaching Hospitals, and Health Systems* (AAMC), 3
Osler, Sir William, 2, 24, 48, 60
Outcomes Project, 3

pancreatitis, 9, 20–21
panic, xiv–xv, 23
Paracelsus, 107
*A Parting Gift* (Sharkey), 129–37
*Passages* (Sheehy), 62, 81
patient-centered care. *See also* doctor-patient relationship
    biopsychosocial model in, 15–16
    empathy in, 8–13
    healing process in, 85
    helplessness in, 16–19, 44–47
    human nature in, 43–45
    IOM and, 2–3
    listening in, 7–8
    nonverbal language in, 45–49
    trust in, 6–8, 48–51
patient-centered interview, xix–xx. *See also* doctor-patient relationship
    A.R.T. paradigm in, 74–79
    assessment in, 76–78
    early moments of, 69–71
    following affect in, 71–72
    observation in, 69–71
    process of, 72–74
    ranking in, 78
    strategies in, 79–85
    transition in, 78–79
*Patient Interviewing: The Human Dimension* (Reiser and Schroder), 56, 74
patient-physician relationship. *See* doctor-patient relationship
penicillin, 112
person-level factors
    in biopsychosocial model, 33–38, 35*f*
    in curing and healing, 107–11
    experience of illness and, 95–99
    style in, 59
    Type A personality in, 48–51
pharmacogenomics, 14
physical appearance, 80
physician burnout, 59, 110
pneumonia, 111–13
polyuria, 17
principles of medicine
    acceptance in, 5–8, 21–24
    competence in, 20–24
    conceptualization in, 13–20
    empathy in, 8–13
    summary on, 24
privilege, of physician, 139
"problem patients," 83–84, 87, 97, 100, 104–5
prophylactic steroids, 23
Psychiatric Aspects of Medical Practice, xix
psychodynamics, 49–51
psychological counseling, xvi, 89
psychosocial framework, 28–29

Ray, Stephen, 5
reductionism, 27–29, 66, 125
*Re-humanizing Medicine* (Kopacz), 101
Reiser, David, xi–xii, xix, 1–2, 56, 74, 89
relationships, in illness, 99–100. *See also* doctor-patient relationship
reorganization, illness and, 92–95
responsibility, medical students and, 59–60
Rogers, Carl, 82
Roosevelt, Franklin Delano, 93
Roosevelt, Theodore, 81
Rosen, David H., xi–xii, 1–2, 93, 99, 102
Rosenman, Ray, 48

Schmale, Art, 46, 98
Schroder, Andrea, 56, 74, 89
*Seasons of a Man's Life* (Levinson), 81
self-awareness, 7, 24, 92–94
   in illness, 100
   meditation and, 19, 81, 110–11, 120, 125
self-compassion, 81
sexual intimacy, 7
shamanism, 67, 121
Sharkey, Frances, 129–37
Shaw, Bernard, 121
Sheehy, Gale, 62, 81
Shelley, Percy B., 116
silence, 6–7, 82, 117
*The Silken Tent* (Frost), 15, 24
sincerity, 13, 80, 84, 125, 129
slang, 65–66
Smith, Robert C., 79
social reciprocity, 6–7
social services, 20–21, 112
spirituality, 19–20
   existential quest and, 126–29
   and healing, 111, 120, 123–26
Still Face Experiment, 6
suffering, death and, 66–67
suicide, 141–42
   obesity and, 60–61, 64
   of physicians, 81

Sullivan, Harry Stack, 62
systems hierarchy, 13–14, 19–20
   biomedical model in, 27–29
   biopsychosocial model in, 29–31, 30$f$, 31$f$
   molecular substance in, 30–31, 30$f$, 31$f$
   stable configuration of, 29
   stages of illness and, 87–89

TED Talk, 66, 84
Thomas, Lewis, 121, 122
*To Err Is Human: Building a Safer Health System* (IOM), 2
touch, in healing, 120–23
transference, 64–65
*Transforming Depression: Healing the Soul through Creativity* (Rosen), 102
Tronick, Edward, 6
trust, 6–8
   in care of Type A patient, 48–51
Tsu, Vivian, 99, 102
Type A personality, 48–51

University of California
   Los Angeles, xii–xiii
   San Francisco, xix
University of Rochester, 5
*The Use of Complementary and Alternative Medicine in United States*, 110–11

Vaillant, George E., 62
Valium, 89
ventricular fibrillation, 35–38, 40$f$–41$f$
Veterans Affairs hospital, 65
visualization, in healing, 116–20

Weil, Andrew, ix, 20
Weiss, Paul, 29
Whitman, Walt, 129
witch doctors, 67

www.ingramcontent.com/pod-product-compliance
Ingram Content Group UK Ltd.
Pitfield, Milton Keynes, MK11 3LW, UK
UKHW021320180426
11947UKWH00015B/1342